The Impact of Patient-Centered Care

Hailun Liang

The Impact of Patient-Centered Care

Promoting Chronic Conditions Management for Older People

Springer

Hailun Liang
Renmin University of China
Beijing, China

ISBN 978-981-16-3967-8 ISBN 978-981-16-3968-5 (eBook)
https://doi.org/10.1007/978-981-16-3968-5

This Springer imprint is published by the registered company Springer Nature Singapore Pte Ltd.
The registered company address is: 152 Beach Road, #21-01/04 Gateway East, Singapore 189721, Singapore

About This Book

The world has experienced a demographic change in the distribution of population toward older ages. At the same time, the global burden of disease is shifting from infectious diseases to non-communicable diseases. Chronic conditions are the leading cause of death and disability globally. The objective of this study is to investigate the impact of patient-centered care (PCC) for older adults with chronic conditions and to add evidence of its effects on the process of care and health outcomes.

Our study reveals significant associations between the status of the PCC and the receipt of preventive care services, cancer care as well as perceiving good health status. The elderly chronic disease patients who have the PCC were more likely to receive preventive screenings and health education and to perceive good physical and mental health status. Our findings suggest that the PCC demonstrates the potential to improve preventive care delivery and health outcomes for the vulnerable older adults with chronic conditions. This work was supported by National Natural Science Foundation of China (grant number: 71804183).

Contents

1 Backgroud of Patient-Centered Care 1
1.1 Background 1
1.2 Significance of Patient-Centered Care 2
1.3 Overview of the Book 3
References 3

2 Theoretical Foundation of Patient-Centered Care 7
2.1 Definitions and Attributes of Patient-Centered Care 7
References 12

3 Conceptual Framework of Patient-Centered Care 15
3.1 Conceptual Framework of Patient-Centered Care 15
3.2 National Accreditation and Recognition PCMH Programs 18
3.3 States' PCMH Programs 22
3.4 Other PCC Interventions and Associated Outcomes 22
3.5 The Evaluation of Patient-Centered Care 24
3.5.1 The Core Areas of PCC Measures 24
3.5.2 Evaluation Design Considerations 26
3.5.3 Main Data Source 27
References 27

4 Patient-Centered Care and Elderly Healthcare 31
4.1 Patient-Centered Care on Older Adults with Chronic Conditions 31
4.2 Conceptual Framework for Evluation 32
4.3 Study Aims and Research Questions 33
4.3.1 Study Objectives 33
4.3.2 Specific Aims 33
4.3.3 Hypotheses 34
4.4 Data and Sample 34
4.4.1 Medical Expenditure Panel Survey 34
4.4.2 Sample Size and Power 35
4.4.3 Strategies for Addressing Missing Values 36

4.5 Measures 38
4.5.1 Independent Variables 38
4.5.2 Dependent Variables 42
4.5.3 Covariates 44
4.6 Sample Weights and Variance Structure 44
4.7 Analysis 47
References 48

5 The Impact of Patient-Centered Care on Preventive Service 51
5.1 Introduction 51
5.2 Demographic and Institutional Characteristics 51
5.3 Bivariate Results 55
5.4 Multivariate Results 58
5.4.1 Multivariate Analysis: PCC Status Associated with Preventive Screening and Health Education 58
5.4.2 PCC Attributes Associated with Receiving Preventive Screening and Health Education 66
References 74

6 The Impact of Patient-Centered Care on Healthcare Outcomes 75
6.1 Introduction 75
6.2 Bivariate Results 75
6.3 Multivariate Results 76
6.3.1 Multivariate Analysis: PCC Status Associated with Health Outcomes 76
6.3.2 Multivariate Analysis: PCC Attributes Associated with Health Outcomes 77

7 The Patient-Centered Care on Cancer Prevention and Treatment 87
7.1 Introduction 87
7.2 The Patient-Centered Oncology Care 88
7.3 Evidence Synthesis 90
7.4 Evidence on the Patient-Centered Oncology Care on Healthcare Utilization and Cost 97
7.5 The Impact of Patient-Centered Oncology Care on Healthcare Utilization and Cost 101
7.6 Practice Implications 103
References 105

8 Policy Implications and Discussions 109
8.1 Introduction 109
8.2 Summary of the Key Findings 110
8.3 Discussions of Findings and Policy Implications 111
8.3.1 Discussion for the Aim 1: Patient-Centered Care and Preventive Care Services 111

8.3.2 Discussion for the Aim 2: Patient-Centered Care and Health Outcome Measures 114
8.4 Overall Impact of the Findings 116
8.4.1 The Implications for Older Adults with Chronic Conditions 116
8.4.2 Implications from the Comparison Between Our Findings with Literature 118
8.4.3 The Generalizability of the Research Findings and Policy Implications 119
8.5 Study Limitations 120
References 121

9 Conclusion 125
References 127

Acronyms

AAAHC	Accreditation Association for Ambulatory Healthcare
AAFP	American Academy of Family Physicians
AAP	American Academy of Pediatrics
ACA	Patient Protection and Affordable Care Act
ACP	American College of Physicians
ADLs	Activities of Daily Living
AHRQ	Agency for Healthcare Research and Quality
AOA	American Osteopathic Association
BPHC	Bureau of Primary Health Care
CAPI	Computer-Assisted Personal Interviewing
CCM	Chronic Care Model
CDC	Centers for Disease Control and Prevention
CMS	Centers for Medicare and Medicaid Services
CPT	Current Procedural Terminology
EFA	Exploratory Factor Analysis
EHR	Electronic Medical Record
FQHC	Federally Qualified Health Centers
HHS	Department of Health and Human Services
HIE	Health Information Exchange
HRSA	Health Resources Services Administration
IADLs	Instrumental Activities of Daily Living
IAPO	International Alliance of Patients' Organizations
IOM	Institute of Medicine
IT	Information Technology
MEPS	Medical Expenditure Panel Survey
NCQA	National Committee for Quality Assurance
NHIS	National Health Interview Survey
OR	Odds Ratio
PCC	Patient-Centered Care
PCMH	Patient-Centered Medical Home
PSUs	Primary Sampling Units
SES	Socioeconomic Status

URAC	Utilization Review Accreditation Committee
USC	Usual Source of Care
USPSTF	U.S. Preventive Services Task Force
VHA	Veterans Health Administration
VIF	Variance Inflation Factor

List of Figures

Fig. 4.1 Conceptual framework of the study. *Source* Donabedian (1988) 32
Fig. 4.2 Analytic samples 37
Fig. 7.1 Conceptual framework for patient-centered oncology care. *Note* The framework is adapted from the Joint Principles of the PCMH (PCPPC, 2012), and Wender and Altshuler (2009) 91
Fig. 7.2 Screening process for the eligible studies 93
Fig. 7.3 Forest plot of effect sizes of ED visit. *Note* 1. A random-effects meta-analysis was used to incorporate heterogeneity among studies. 2. The direction of effect: the negative results indicate that an intervention works in reducing ER visits. 3. Colligan et al. (2017a, 2017b) were associated with the community oncology medical home (COME HOME) model; Goyal et al. (2014) and Kohler et al. (2015) were associated with the PCMH program of Community Care of North Carolina (CCNC) 99
Fig. 7.4 Funnel plot of effect sizes of ED visits. *Note* Results of the Egger's test: t = 0.288, $p = 0.80$ 99
Fig. 7.5 Forest plot of effect sizes of hospitalizations. *Note* 1. A random-effects meta-analysis was used to incorporate heterogeneity among studies. 2. The direction of effect: the negative results indicate that an intervention works in reducing hospitalizations. 3. Colligan et al. (2017a, 2017b) were associated with the community oncology medical home (COME HOME) model; Goyal et al. (2014) and Kohler et al. (2015) were associated with the PCMH program of Community Care of North Carolina (CCNC) 100
Fig. 7.6 Funnel plot of effect sizes of hospitalizations. *Note* Results of the Egger's test: t = 0.835, $p = 0.491$ 101

List of Tables

Table 2.1 Overview of definitions, core components and features of patient-centered care . . . 9
Table 2.2 Attributes of patient-centered care . . . 11
Table 3.1 Features of national accreditation and recognition programs . . . 20
Table 3.2 Summary of PCC interventions in empirical studies . . . 25
Table 4.1 Sample frames by year and by panel, MEPS 2009–2013 . . . 35
Table 4.2 Sensitivity analyses: weighted analytic samples compared to excluded samples . . . 38
Table 4.3 MEPS items used for measuring patient-centered care attributes . . . 40
Table 4.4 Factor loading of patient-centered care measures . . . 41
Table 4.5 Patient-centered care status and samples . . . 42
Table 4.6 Description and inclusion criteria for each screening measure . . . 43
Table 4.7 Description for each covariate . . . 45
Table 4.8 Weighted dependent variables by year, 2009–2013 . . . 46
Table 5.1 Sociodemographic and health characteristics: 2009–2013 US Civilian Noninstitutionalized Population Age 65 and above with chronic condition . . . 52
Table 5.2 Preventive care and health education rates: comparisons between patient-centered care patients and non patient-centered care patients . . . 56
Table 5.3 Multivariate analysis of correlates of preventive care and health education rates . . . 59
Table 5.4 Multivariate analysis of correlates of PCC attributes with preventive care and health education rates . . . 67
Table 6.1 Multivariate analysis of correlates of health status and adverse utilization events . . . 78
Table 6.2 Multivariate analysis of correlates of PCC attributes with health status and adverse event . . . 82

Table 6.3 Health status and adverse events: comparisons between patient-centered care patients and non patient-centered care patients 86
Table 7.1 Study characteristics 94

Chapter 1
Backgroud of Patient-Centered Care

1.1 Background

Chronic conditions are the leading cause of death and disability in the United States (Centers for Disease Control and Prevention, 2013), and also the major contributor to the growth of healthcare spending (Gerteis et al., 2014; Paez et al., 2009). As of 2012, about half of all adults—117 million people—had one or more chronic health conditions. One of four adults had two or more chronic health conditions (Ward et al., 2014). Chronic illnesses are conditions that last a year or more and require ongoing medical attention and/or limit activities of daily living (Warshaw, 2006), for example, arthritis, asthma, chronic respiratory conditions, diabetes, heart disease, human immunodeficiency virus infection, and hypertension. In addition to these physical medical conditions, chronic conditions also comprise conditions such as substance use addictions, dementia and other cognitive disorders and disabilities.

In terms of the rate of multiple chronic conditions, the prevalence is raised with the age increasing, and is considerably higher among older adults. The risks, such as unnecessary hospitalizations, duplicative medication, conflicting medical advice, impairment functional status and mortality, are also raised with the increasing number of chronic conditions that a patient has (Anderson, 2010; Lee, et al., 2007; Vogeli, et al., 2007; Warshaw, 2006; Wolff, et al., 2002). This situation is even more complicated when the synergistic interactions occur due to the combinations of multiple conditions, for example, the co-occurrences of serious mental illnesses with serious medical illness (Wolff, et al., 2002).

At the same time, the required resources for chronic conditions management are enormous. In term of Medicare program, the increased spending on managing chronic diseases has become one of the key factors that drive the overall medical expense growth (Thorpe et al., 2010). Patients with chronic conditions are facing considerable challenges related to higher costs in prescription drugs and total out-of-pocket costs (Anderson, 2010).

In addition, the combined impact of population aging seriously increase the challenges of managing chronic conditions among the burgeoning population. Although

H. Liang, *The Impact of Patient-Centered Care*,
https://doi.org/10.1007/978-981-16-3968-5_1

evaluations on quality and cost of chronic care have been carried out, insufficient attention has been paid to the older adults to meet longer-term needs of those with chronic conditions.

1.2 Significance of Patient-Centered Care

The greatest challenge in healthcare is to provide optimal care for older adults with chronic conditions and comorbidities. Older adults with chronic conditions are very heterogeneous in health status, disease severity, treatment options, prognosis and risk of adverse events (Boyd & Fortin, 2011; Boyd et al., 2005; Institute of Medicine, 2001). Existing literature suggests that the optimal management of chronic conditions depends highly on active involvement of the patients (Holman & Lorig, 2000; Tsai et al., 2010). The concept of patient-centered care (PCC) has become an essential component in the healthcare sector since the 1950s (Bauman et al., 2003). PCC is principally described as an effective approach to deliver care that meets the specific needs, values, and beliefs of patients (Institute of Medicine, 2001). A significant increase in its popularity starts to emerge over the past 15 years, presumably because primary care systems are seeking solutions to the cope with the challenges from the population aging and significant burden of chronic conditons.

In 2007, the American Academy of Pediatrics (AAP) joined with the American Academy of Family Physicians (AAFP), the American College of Physicians (ACP), and the American Osteopathic Association (AOA) relased the Joint Principles of the Patient Centered Medical Home (PCMH or medical home), which is generally described as a model or philosophy of patient-centered care, that encourages providers and care teams to meet patients where they are, from the most simple to the most complex conditions (AAFP et al., 2007; Patient-Centered Primary Care Collaborative, 2009). Additionally, the PCMH model focuses on chronic condtion management, shared decision making with patients, enhanced access, and coordination with community-based services (Weedon et al., 2012).

The PCMH draws on principles from the well-known Wagner's Chronic Care Model (CCM), which highlights self-management support, decision support, delivery system design, clinical information systems, healthcare organization, and community resources (Bodenheimer et al., 2002; Coleman et al., 2009; Wagner et al., 1996a, 1996b, 1999, 2001). By applying CCM, PCC has become a widely accepted model that direct the delivery of high-quality and safe care targeted to address the increasing health demands of aging population with chronic conditions (Luxford et al., 2010).

Although PCC has been theoretically conceived being able to overcome current challenges from fragmentation and poor coordination of care, it is unclear whether the model is appropriate for deliveing chronic care to aged patients with high-risk or complex healthcare needs. Futher investigations are need to tailor PCC model according to the needs of specific patient population, the nature of their diseases, and other predisposing or enabling factors (Stevens et al., 2010).

There is growing interest in exploring the impact of PCC on various outcomes, but little is known about its effectiveness for delivering chronic care to older adultes. It is unclear which attributes of PCC are required for aging population's chronic care and whether the model will enhance patient perceived satisfaction, health outcomes, safety, and efficiency (Boult & Wieland, 2010).

1.3 Overview of the Book

The objective of this book is to investigate the impact of PCC for older adults with chronic conditions, and to add evidence of its effects on patient's experiences, process of care, and health outcomes. The specific aims of this book are to: (1) assess the association between the receipt of PCC and chronic disease management among older adults, measured by the receipt of preventive screening and health education for chronic diseases, as well as cancer care; and (2) assess the association between the receipt of PCC and chronic disease health outcomes among older adults, measured by patient perceived health status and incidence of adverse utilization events.

In pursing the aims, this book evaluates the associations between the receipt of PCC and healthcare process as well as outcome measures. This book is organized into nine chapters. The first chapter provides an introduction and background to the book. It describes briefly the background and the rationale of conducting this study. The second chapter investigates the theoretical foundation of PCC. Chapter Three describes the conceptual framework of PCC. Chapter Four reports PCC and elderly healthcare. Chapter Five, Six and Seven investigate the impact of PCC on Preventive Services Provision, health outcomes and oncology care. Chapter Eight and Nine summarizes the policy implications, discussions and conclusions of this work.

References

American Academy of Family Physicians (AAFP), American Academy of Pediatrics (AAP), American College of Physicians (ACP), et al. (2007). *Joint principles of the patient-centered medical home*. Accessed on January 8, 2016. Available at: www.aafp.org/online/etc/medialib/aafp_org/documents/policy/fed/jointprinciplespcmh0207.Par.0001.File.dat/022107medicalhome.pdf.

Anderson G. (2010). Chronic care: making the case for ongoing care. Accessed on January 8, 2016. Available at: http://www.rwjf.org/files/research/50968chronic.care.chartbook.pdf.

Bauman, A. E., Fardy, H. J., & Harris, P. G. (2003). Getting it right: Why bother with patient-centred care? *Medical Journal of Australia, 179*(5), 253–256.

Bodenheimer, T., Wagner, E. H., & Grumbach, K. (2002). Improving primary care for patients with chronic illness: The chronic care model, Part 2. *JAMA, 288*(15), 1909–1914.

Boult, C., & Wieland, G. D. (2010). Comprehensive primary care for older patients with multiple chronic conditions: "Nobody rushes you through" . *JAMA, 304*(17), 1936–1943.

Boyd, C. M., Darer, J., Boult, C., Fried, L. P., Boult, L., & Wu, A. W. (2005). Clinical practice guidelines and quality of care for older patients with multiple comorbid diseases: Implications for pay for performance. *JAMA, 294*(6), 716–724.

Boyd, C. M., & Fortin, M. (2011). Future of multimorbidity research: How should understanding of multimorbidity inform health system design? *Public Health Reviews, 32*, 451–474.

Centers for Disease Control and Prevention. (2013a). Summary Health Statistics for the U.S. Population: National Health Interview Survey, 2012. Accessed on January 8, 2016. Available at: http://www.cdc.gov/nchs/data/series/sr_10/sr10_259.pdf.

Coleman, K., Austin, B. T., Brach, C., & Wagner, E. H. (2009). Evidence on the chronic care model in the new millennium. *Health Affairs (Millwood), 28*(1), 75–85.

Gerteis, J., Izrael, D., et al. (2014). *Multiple chronic conditions chartbook.* Accessed on January 8, 2016. Available at: http://www.ahrq.gov/sites/default/files/wysiwyg/professionals/prevention-chronic-care/decision/mcc/mccchartbook.pdf.

Holman, H., & Lorig, K. (2000). Patients as partners in managing chronic disease. Partnership is a prerequisite for effective and efficient health care. *BMJ, 320*(7234), 526–527.

Institute of Medicine. (2001). *Crossing the quality chasm: A new health system for the 21st century.* Accessed on January 8, 2016. Available at: www.nap.edu/.../quality_chasm/reportbrief.pdf.

Lee, T. A., Shields, A. E., Vogeli, C., Gibson, T. B., Woong-Sohn, M., Marder, W. D., Blumenthal, D., & Weiss, K. B. (2007). Mortality rate in veterans with multiple chronic conditions. *Journal of General Internal Medicine, 22*(Suppl 3), 403–407.

Luxford, K., Piper, D., Dunbar, N., & Poole, N. (2010). *Patient-centered care: Improving quality and safety by focusing care on patients and consumers—Discussion paper*. Accessed on January 8, 2016. Available at: http://www.safetyandquality.gov.au/wp-content/uploads/2012/01/PCCC-DiscussPaper.pdf.

Paez, K. A., Zhao, L., & Hwang, W. (2009). Rising out-of-pocket spending for chronic conditions: A ten-year trend. *Health Affairs (Millwood), 28*(1), 15–25.

Patient-Centered Primary Care Collaborative. (2009). *Proof in practice. A compilation of patient centered medical home pilot and demonstration projects.* Accessed on January 8, 2016. Available at: https://www.pcpcc.org/sites/default/files/media/PilotGuidePip.pdf.

Stevens, G. D., Pickering, T. A., & Laqui, S. A. (2010). Relationship of medical home quality with school engagement and after-school participation among children with asthma. *Journal of Asthma, 47*(9), 1001–1010.

Thorpe, K. E., Ogden, L. L., & Galactionova, K. (2010). Chronic conditions account for rise in Medicare spending from 1987 to 2006. *Health Affairs (Millwood), 29*(4), 718–724.

Tsai, J., Shi, L., Yu, W. L., & Lebrun, L. A. (2010). Usual source of care and the quality of medical care experiences: A cross-sectional survey of patients from a Taiwanese community. *Medical Care, 48*(7), 628–634.

Vogeli, C., Shields, A. E., Lee, T. A., Gibson, T. B., Marder, W. D., Weiss, K. B., & Blumenthal, D. (2007). Multiple chronic conditions: Prevalence, health consequences, and implications for quality, care management, and costs. *Journal of General Internal Medicine, 22*(Suppl 3), 391–395.

Wagner, E. H., Austin, B. T., & Von Korff, M. (1996a). Improving outcomes in chronic illness. *Managed Care Quarterly, 4*(2), 12–25.

Wagner, E. H., Austin, B. T., & Von Korff, M. (1996b). Organizing care for patients with chronic illness. *Milbank Quarterly, 74*(4), 511–544.

Wagner, E. H., Davis, C., Schaefer, J., Von Korff, M., & Austin, B. (1999). A survey of leading chronic disease management programs: Are they consistent with the literature? *Managed Care Quarterly, 7*(3), 56–66.

Wagner, E. H., Glasgow, R. E., Davis, C., Bonomi, A. E., Provost, L., McCulloch, D., Carver, P., & Sixta, C. (2001). Quality improvement in chronic illness care: A collaborative approach. *Joint Commission Journal on Quality Improvement, 27*(2), 63–80.

Warshaw, G. (2006). Introduction: Advances and challenges in care of older people with chronic illness. *Generation, 30*(3), 5–10.

Ward, B. W., Schiller, J. S., & Goodman, R. A. (2014). Multiple chronic conditions among US adults: A 2012 update. *Preventing Chronic Disease, 11*, E62.

Weedon, D., Carbone, P., Bilder, D., O'Brien, S., & Dorius, J. (2012). Building a person-centered medical home: Lessons from a program for people with developmental disabilities. *Journal of Health Care for the Poor and Underserved, 23*(4), 1600–1608.

Wolff, J. L., Starfield, B., & Anderson, G. (2002). Prevalence, expenditures, and complications of multiple chronic conditions in the elderly. *Archives of Internal Medicine, 162*(20), 2269–2276.

Chapter 2
Theoretical Foundation of Patient-Centered Care

2.1 Definitions and Attributes of Patient-Centered Care

The concept of PCC has become an essetial component in the healthcare sector since the 1950s (Bauman et al., 2003). A significant increase in its popularity starts to emerge over the past 15 years, presumably because primary care systems are seeking solutions to the cope with the challenges from the population aging and significant burden of chronic conditons. PCC is pricipally described as an effective approach to deliver care that meets the specific needs, values, and beliefs of patients (Institute of Medicine, 2001). PCC has become a widely accepted model that direct the delivery of high-quality and safe care targeted to address the increasing health demands of aging population with chronic conditions (Luxford et al., 2010).

The IOM defines PCC as healthcare that establishes a partnership among practitioners, patients, and their families (when appropriate) to ensure that decisions respect patients' wants, needs, and preferences and that patients have the education and support they need to make decisions and participate in their own care (Institute of Medicine, 2001). Based on this definition, Alliance for Home Health Quality and Innovation summarized the definition into four core components as "whole person" care, comprehensive communication and coordination, patient support and empowerment, and ready access (Alliance for Home Health Quality and Innovation, 2013). In 2002, to help patients and their healthcare providers make better decisions, the Agency for Healthcare Research and Quality (AHRQ) defined the PCC as follows: patients become active participants in their own care and receive services designed to focus on their individual needs and preferences, in addition to advice and counsel from health professionals. They also developed a series of tools to help determine treatment preferences (AHRQ, 2002). The International Alliance of Patients' Organizations (IAPO) states that the essence of patient-centered healthcare is that the healthcare system is designed and delivered to address the healthcare needs and preferences of patients so that healthcare is appropriate and cost-effective. The IAPO's declaration sets out five principles of patient-centered healthcare: respect; choice and empowerment; patient involvement in health policy; access and support and

H. Liang, *The Impact of Patient-Centered Care*,
https://doi.org/10.1007/978-981-16-3968-5_2

information (IAPO, 2006). The Picker Institute is an independent non-profit organization dedicated to advancing principles of PCC. The Picker Institute identifies seven dimensions of PCC: (1) respect for patients' values, preferences and expressed needs; (2) coordination of care and integration of services within an institutional setting; (3) communication between patient and providers; dissemination of accurate, timely and appropriate information; and education about the long-term implications of disease and illness; (4) physical care, comfort and the alleviation of pain; (5) emotional support and alleviation of fears and anxiety; (6) involvement of family and friends; and (7) transition and continuity from one locus of care to another (Gerteis, 1993).

Besides these definitions of PCC, such concepts and dimensions of PCC can be drawn from the description of patient-centered medical home (PCMH). The American Academy of Pediatrics introduced the medical home concept in 1967. A generation later, in 2004 the specialty of family medicine called for all patients to have a "personal medical home." In 2003 National Committee for Quality Assurance (NCQA) launched Physician Practice Connections, a PCMH precursor program. In 2007, the American Academy of Family Physicians, American Academy of Pediatrics, American College of Physicians, and American Osteopathic Association released Joint PCMH Principles. In 2008, NCQA launched the first PCMH Recognition program. Based on the recognition standard of NCQA, PCC can be defined as: healthcare that strengthens the physician–patient relationship by replacing episodic care with coordinated care and a long-term healing relationship (NCQA, 2014). Table 2.1 show the comparison among these definitions and their core components and features.

PCC remains insufficiently understood and is described by varied terminology with different meanings (Bauman et al., 2003; Mead & Bower, 2000, 2002; Stewart, 2001). Concepts such as person-centered care, individual-centered care, or family-centered care are used inconsistently, leading to barriers and confusion in practice and research. In order to address the confusion, several conceptual analyses have been conducted to synthesize the evidence to inform the key component of PCC (Hughes et al., 2008; Leplege et al., 2007; McCormack & McCance, 2006). However, most reviews failed to draw solid conclusions on whether patient-centered care has positive impacts on health outcomes for patients with chronic disease, neither particular on older adults. In a recent study of PCC, it was discussed that the future studies should focus the specific dimensions of PCC and how its impact on specific targeted population or conditions (Rathert et al., 2013).

In this book, we summarized the multiple definitions and frameworkd above and found there were many overlapping elements among different frameworks developed to describe the key attributes of PCC. By comparing these existing definitions of PCC, we found that the definition from IOM is the origin and basis for many other definitions devloped by other organizations. Besides, this definition and its dimensions of PCC are targeted to primary care settings. In terms of the other definitions, the definition from IAPO is developed with strong patients' and patient organizations' voice. The definition from Picker Institute focuses on healthcare providers, that is, a patient-centered approach must also address the medical providers' experience, the reason it that providers' ability and inclination to deliver effectively care for patients is unquestionably compromised if they do not feel cared for themselves.

Table 2.1 Overview of definitions, core components and features of patient-centered care

Organization	Definitions	Core components/domains	Features
Institute of Medicine (IOM) (2001)	Healthcare that establishes a partnership among practitioners, patients, and their families (when appropriate) to ensure that decisions respect patients' wants, needs, and preferences and that patients have the education and support they need to make decisions and participate in their own care	"Whole person" care; comprehensive communication and coordination; patient support and empowerment; and ready access	The definition and dimensions were targeted and originally applied to primary care settings
Agency for Healthcare Research and Quality (AHRQ) (2002, 2010)	Patients become active participants in their own care and receive services designed to focus on their individual needs and preferences, in addition to advice and counsel from health professionals	A patient-centered orientation; comprehensive, team-based care; care that is coordinated; superb access to care; a systems-based approach to quality and safety	The five components are drawn on the concept of the PCMH, in which a practice is organized to provide truly coordinated, proactive and therefore cost-effective care (AHRQ, 2010)
The International Alliance of Patients' Organizations (IAPO) (2006)	Healthcare system is designed and delivered to address the healthcare needs and preferences of patients so that healthcare is appropriate and cost-effective	Respect; choice and empowerment; patient involvement in health policy; access and support and information	The principles were developed with strong patients' and patient organizations' voice

(continued)

Table 2.1 (continued)

Organization	Definitions	Core components/domains	Features
Picker Institute (2008)	Patient-centered care is a model in which providers develop partnership with patients and their families to identify and satisfy the full range of patient needs and preferences, while simultaneously supporting the professional and personal aspirations of their staff	Respect for patients' values, preferences and expressed needs; coordination of care and integration of services within an institutional setting; communication between patient and providers; dissemination of accurate, timely and appropriate information; and education about the long-term implications of disease and illness; physical care, comfort and the alleviation of pain; emotional support and alleviation of fears and anxiety; involvement of family and friends; and transition and continuity from one locus of care to another	This definition also focuses on staff. To succeed, a patient-centered approach must also address the staff experience, as staff's ability and inclination to effectively care for patients is unquestionably compromised if they do not feel cared for themselves
National Committee for Quality Assurance (NCQA) (2008)	Healthcare that strengthens the physician–patient relationship by replacing episodic care with coordinated care and a long-term healing relationship	Access and communication; patient tracking and registry functions; care management; patient self-management and support; electronic prescribing; test tracking; referral tracking; performance reporting and improvement, and advanced electronic communication	These dimensions are more specific and operationalized, as they are drawn from the standard of PCMH recognition

Table 2.2 Attributes of patient-centered care

The main attributes of PCC emerges from synergy among the above definitions
• Whole person care orientation
• Patient engagement in care
• Enhanced access to care

The definitions from NCQA and AHRQ are drawn from the recognition standards of the PCMH, thus these dimensions are more specific and operationalized.

Clearly, there are also substantial commonality of key attribute across the varying definitions and frameworks summarized above. By reviewing these definitions and frameworks, we synthesized the following three main atrribues of PCC embeded in the most of definitions described above. These attributes are principally consistent with the body of studies that has previously investigated PCC on an empirical basis (Aysola et al., 2013; Beal et al., 2009; Jones et al., 2015). Table 2.2 shows the three atrribues of PCC.

a. Whole person care orientation

From the patient's perspective, this attribute of PCC means that each patient has a usual source of care, which is having an ongoing relationship with a personal physician whose role is in total care for the patient. From the provider's perspective, the physician is responsible for providing first contact, continuous and comprehensive care for patient's healthcare needs and taking responsibility for appropriately coordinating care with other healthcare professionals. This includes acute care, chronic care, preventive services, community services and supports, and referral services to the other providers.

b. Patient engagement in care

Patients who actively participate in their own care are more likely to manage their conditions and stay healthy through obtaining more information regarding their health problems, adhering treatment, doing physical exercises, having healthy diet, and receiving preventive care services (Hibbard & Cunningham, 2008). At the same time, providers can also benefit from the partnership with patients by knowing patient's medications and medical history well and better coordinating care across all elements of healthcare system. The active patient engagement requires a partnership between patients and their providers, which will ensures that providers respect patients' needs and preferences when they make decisions, or patients can make decisions for their own care with the education and support from their providers.

c. Enhanced access to care

Providers commit to enhancing patients' access to care by timely responding to patient's health needs and accommodating healthcare for patients. By applying personnel, systems and infrastructure investment, such as expanded hours, open scheduling, and new methods for patient-physician communication, patients will be able to get timely access to care, after hours care service, 24/7 telephone or email access, and improved communication via health IT innovations.

References

Agency for Healthcare Research and Quality. (2002). *Expanding patient-centered care to empower patients and assist providers*. Accessed on January 8, 2016. Available at: http://www.ahrq.gov/research/findings/factsheets/patient-centered/ria-issue5/index.html.

Agency for Healthcare Research and Quality. (2010). *Medical home definition*. Accessed on January 8, 2016. Available at: http://pcmh.ahrq.gov/sites/default/files/attachments/Strategies%20to%20Put%20Patients%20at%20the%20Center%20of%20Primary%20Care.pdf.

Alliance for Home Health Quality and Innovation. (2013). *Patient & family engagement across the care continuum*. Accessed on January 8, 2016. Available at: http://ahhqi.org/images/uploads/NPWF_Presentation_-_Alliance_for_Home_Health_Quality_and_Innovation_(September_2013).pdf.

Aysola, J., Bitton, A., Zaslavsky, A. M., & Ayanian, J. Z. (2013). Quality and equity of primary care with patient-centered medical homes: Results from a national survey. *Medical Care, 51*(1), 68–77.

Bauman, A. E., Fardy, H. J., & Harris, P. G. (2003). Getting it right: Why bother with patient-centred care? *Medical Journal of Australia, 179*(5), 253–256.

Beal, A., Hernandez, S., & Doty, M. (2009). Latino access to the patient-centered medical home. *Journal of General Internal Medicine, 24*(Suppl 3), 514–520.

Gerteis, M., Edgman-Levitan, S., Walker, J. D., Stoke, D. M., Cleary, P. D., & Delbanco, T. L. (1993). What patients really want. *Health Management Quarterly, 15*(3), 2–6.

Hibbard, J. H., & Cunningham, P. J. (2008). *How engaged are consumers in their health and health care, and why does it matter*? Accessed on January 8, 2016. Available at: http://www.hschange.com/CONTENT/1019/1019.pdf.

Hughes, J. C., Bamford, C., & May, C. (2008). Types of centredness in health care: Themes and concepts. *Medicine, Health Care and Philosophy, 11*(4), 455–463.

Institute of Medicine. (2001). *Crossing the quality chasm: A new health system for the 21st century*. Accessed on January 8, 2016. Available at: www.nap.edu/.../quality_chasm/reportbrief.pdf.

International Alliance of Patients' Organizations. (2006). *Declaration on patient-centred healthcare*. Accessed on January 8, 2016. Available at: http://iapo.org.uk/sites/default/filesfiles/IAPO%20Declaration%20on%20Patient-Centred%20Healthcare%20Poster.pdf.

Jones, A. L., Cochran, S. D., Leibowitz, A., Wells, K. B., Kominski, G., & Mays, V. M. (2015). Usual primary care provider characteristics of a patient-centered medical home and mental health service use. *Journal of General Internal Medicine, 30*(12), 1828–1836.

Leplege, A., Gzil, F., Cammelli, M., Lefeve, C., Pachoud, B., & Ville, I. (2007). Person-centredness: Conceptual and historical perspectives. *Disability and Rehabilitation, 29*(20–21), 1555–1565.

Luxford, K., Piper, D., Dunbar, N., & Poole, N. (2010). *Patient-centered care: Improving quality and safety by focusing care on patients and consumers—Discussion paper*. Accessed on January 8, 2016. Available at: http://www.safetyandquality.gov.au/wp-content/uploads/2012/01/PCCC-DiscussPaper.pdf.

McCormack, B., & McCance, T. V. (2006). Development of a framework for person-centred nursing. *Journal of Advanced Nursing, 56*(5), 472–479.

Mead, N., & Bower, P. (2000). Patient-centredness: A conceptual framework and review of the empirical literature. *Social Science and Medicine, 51*(7), 1087–1110.

Mead, N., & Bower, P. (2002). Patient-centred consultations and outcomes in primary care: A review of the literature. *Patient Education and Counseling, 48*(1), 51–61.

National Committee for Quality Assurance (NCQA). (2008). *Standards and guidelines for physician practice connections—patient-centered medical home*. Accessed on January 8, 2016. Available at: http://www.ncqa.org/Portals/0/Programs/Recognition/PCMH_Overview_Apr01.pdf.

National Committee for Quality Assurance (NCQA). (2014). *The future of patient-centered medical homes: foundation for a better health care system*. Accessed on January 8, 2016. Available at: http://www.ncqa.org/Portals/0/Public%20Policy/2014%20Comment%20Letters/The_Future_of_PCMH.pdf.

Picker Institute. (2008). *Principles of person centred care*. Accessed on September 1, 2021. Available at: https://www.picker.org/about-us/picker-principles-of-person-centred-care/.

Rathert, C., Wyrwich, M. D., & Boren, S. A. (2013). Patient-centered care and outcomes: A systematic review of the literature. *Medical Care Research and Review, 70*(4), 351–379.

Stewart, M. (2001). Towards a global definition of patient centred care. *BMJ, 322*(7284), 444–445.

Chapter 3
Conceptual Framework of Patient-Centered Care

3.1 Conceptual Framework of Patient-Centered Care

Since the concept of PCC evolved, researchers and policy makers bring together primary care practitioners working on transforming the concept to the real practice. Compared with individual or combined PCC interventions developed and implemented in various empirical studies, PCMH has become a widely accepted model and is being rapidly adopted nationwide with the support from government agencies and professional organizations.

In evolution of the PCMH model, the CCM play an integral role that provides the foundation to revolutionize care from the provider-centered to the patient self-management driven. In 1998, the CCM was created to summarize the essential components for improving chronic care at the community, health systems, patients and practice levels. The CCM includes six components that are hypothesized to have impact on the chronic disease management and furtherly affect patient health outcomes. The six components are (1) community resources and policies, that is, advocating local facilities to improve health care (e.g. developing partnerships with community-based organizations to develop and implement interventions, encourage chronic disease patient to participate in community programs. etc.), (2) health system — organization of health care, that is, preparing the whole health system for the change, and motivate improvement at all levels of healthcare organizations (e.g. facilitating care coordination across different levels of healthcare organizations by developing agreements, etc.), (3) self-management support, that is, engaging patient to manage their health (e.g. healthcare providers and patients working together to define health problems, set healthcare goals, develop care plan and solve problem, etc.), (4) delivery system design, that is, transforming healthcare system to coordinate care delivery processes (e.g. integrating care process and providing chronic condition management services for patients with complex healthcare needs, etc.), (5) decision support, that is, sharing evidence-based information with patients and encourage their participating in decision making (e.g. discussing clinical guidelines with patients and respecting patient's preferences, etc.), and (6) clinical information systems, that is,

H. Liang, *The Impact of Patient-Centered Care*,
https://doi.org/10.1007/978-981-16-3968-5_3

managing patient's healthcare data with information system support (e.g. providing care reminders for patients between two visits, monitoring healthcare performance, etc.) (Wagner et al.,). Each components and in their combination fosters vigorous interactions between the activated patients and prepared providers with resources and expertise, which triggers healthier patients, more satisfied providers, and cost savings (Bodenheimer et al., 2002; Coleman et al., 2009; Wagner et al., 2001). The PCMH draw important elements from the CCM, especially the component of patient self-management and informed empowered patient, to enhance the care coordination and communication, and transform primary care into "what patients want it to be" (NCQA, 2014).

To reach the full potential of PCMH, three aspects of input are inevitable and foundational, that are: health IT, workforce and finance (AHRQ, 2015). In terms of health IT, the use of electronic health record is widely recognized as one of the central elements of PCMH, which support the PCMH on collecting, storing, and measuring patient health data and facilitating population-level evaluation. The implementation of health information exchange (HIE) enable clinical information be shared across multiple care settings, which support the care coordination and reduce the duplicate services. The use of registries, such as for specific diseases, preventive care and procedures, allow for capturing information on which patients have specific conditions, and identifying care gaps for vulnerable sub-populations (Bates & Bitton, 2010). Health IT can also support clinical decision making, patient self-management and communication (AHRQ, 2015). As for the aspect of personnel, a strong primary care workforce is an imperative element of the PCMH. Care delivered through PCMH model by an interdisciplinary team-based system, which calls for a variety of different medical professionals work together with clear performance goals, shared leadership, and effective communication. For the small practice, the key strategies for the team transformation are enhanced training and team communication. The reason is the biggest challenge faced by small practice is lack of workforce. Therefore, the cross-trained health professionals can take multiple roles in a team and the timely ongoing communications among teams will ensure patient's safety and improve efficiency with limited human resources. For the large practices, the main challenges could be the multi-sites management and unifying the care standards across various teams. It requires the development of protocols to support teams meet the unified clinical goals. Finally, with regard to the support of finance, payment reforms are needed to compensate providers for enhanced access, care coordination, and their contributions in reducing duplication across the care continuum. Besides, the multi-payer participation can be used to promote the payment reform through public–private partnerships. These payment reforms should be widely piloted and comprehensively evaluated, and rapidly scaled up for those shown to be effective.

In addition to the infrastructural and personnel input for promoting PCMH, the healthcare policies have created a favorable environment for the PCMH to be tested. Section 3502 of the Patient Protection and Affordable Care Act (ACA) directs the Department of Health and Human Services (HHS) to provide grants to eligible healthcare entities to establish community-based interdisciplinary, inter-professional teams to support primary care practices. The proliferation of public and private medical home pilot projects and demonstrations presents preliminary evidence on PCMH's potentials in improving health outcomes and reducing healthcare cost (Bitton, 2010). At federal level, the HHS announced the Multi-Payer Advanced Primary Care Practice (MAPCP) demonstration program in 2009, which was formally implemented in eight states in 2011 and ran for 3 years. The providers who participated in this program were reimbursed on the fee-for-service basis and with the bonus from states for their transformation to PCMH (HHS, 2012). One of the other demonstration projects, Federally Qualified Health Centers (FQHC) Advanced Primary Care Practice demonstration was operated by the Centers for Medicare and Medicaid Services (CMS) in partnership with the Health Resources Services Administration (HRSA) from 2011 to 2014. A total of 434 FQHC sites involved in and up to 195,000 Medicare patients benefited from the program. The participating FQHCs received care management fee for each Medicare beneficiary on a monthly basis for their receipt of primary care services. The demonstration projects concluded on October 2014, and the evaluation showed the PCMH model can improve quality of care, promote patient health and lower healthcare cost (CMS, 2015). At state level, there were also a number of states, such as Colorado, Oregon, Ohio, Michigan and Pennsylvania, operated state level PCMH pilot projects. Among them, the Pennsylvania Chronic Care Initiative (PCCI) was created to improve diabetes care by involving practice coach and care managers, and using registries and quality reporting. The program showed significant improvement in several diabetes clinical measures, such as HbA1c and related cardiovascular risk factors (Bojadzievski & Gabbay, 2011). In addition to these demonstration projects, there were several private sector PCMH programs, such as the Pennsylvania-based Geisinger Health System PCMH model and the Minnesota-based HealthPartner program. The key features of Geisinger Health System PCMH model included use of an advanced EHR system, a "Personal Health Navigator" aiming to providing 24-7 access, and highly collaborative team-based team (Paulus et al., 2008). A recent Geisinger PCMH study using longitudinal clinic-level claims data showed the longer PCMH exposure is associated with lower acute inpatient admission rates, which was the largest savings component of Geisinger health system's PCMH (Maeng et al., 2015).

With the ongoing support for PCMH demonstration from federal government, state government and health plans, a great number of practices get PCMH recognitions or accreditations. In the next section, we will compare the different national accreditation bodies, private payers and states embracing the PCMH models. Among them, the following national entities stand out among the multitude of accreditation and recognition initiatives.

3.2 National Accreditation and Recognition PCMH Programs

PCMH programs accredited or recognized by the Accreditation Association for Ambulatory Healthcare (AAAHC), the Joint Commission, the National Committee for Quality Assurance (NCQA) and Utilization Review Accreditation Committee (URAC) are national in scope. All these four have published set of standards, which have being applied by a large number of healthcare organizations into their care delivery.

a. NCQA's PCMH recognition

Established in 1990, the NCQA is an independent non-profit organization that works to improve healthcare quality through the administration of evidence-based standards, measures, programs, and accreditation, and it aims building consensus across the industry by working with policy makers, employers, doctors, and patients, as well as health plans. NCQA's PCMH recognition is the first (released in 2008) and the most widely-used formal assessment to transform primary care practices into medical homes (NCQA, 2014). NCQA PCMH 2014 recognition is based on six standards: (1) Patient-centered access: accommodate patients' needs during and after hours, provide medical home information, offer team-based care; (2) Team-based care: engage all practice team members by providing medical home information, meet cultural and linguistic needs of patients and offer team-based care; (3) Population health management: collect and use data for population management; (4) Care management and support: use evidence-based guidelines for preventive, acute and chronic care management; (5) Care coordination and care transitions: track and coordinate tests, referrals and care transitions; (6) Performance measurement and quality improvement: use performance and experience data for continuous improvement (NCQA, 2008,2014).

NCQA recognizes primary care practices that meet the scoring criteria for Level 1, 2, or 3 as assessed against the PCMH requirements. As of November 2014, NCQA reports 8386 practices have received PCMH recognition.

b. AAAHC's medical home accreditation standards

Founded in 1979, AAAHC is a non-profit organization which accredits ambulatory healthcare organizations, including ambulatory surgery centers, office-based surgery centers, endoscopy centers, and college student health centers, as well as health plans, such as health maintenance organizations and preferred provider organizations (Kongstvedt, 2007). In 2009, the AAAHC added the Medical Home to the types of organizations that it accredits. It offers on-site surveys for organizations seeking Medical Home accreditation or certification (AAAHC, 2015). AAAHC's Medical Home Accreditation Standards is based on eight core standards and 19 adjunct standards. The eight core standards are: (1) Patient rights and responsibilities; (2) Governance; (3) Administration; (4) Quality of care; (5) Quality management and improvement; (6) Clinical records and health information; (7) Infection prevention control and safety; (8) Facilities and environment (AAAHC, 2015).

AAAHC's recognition program involves 238 items, which is the highest number of assessment survey compared with other programs. AAAHC provides two options to applicants, which are either "accreditation" (obtaining base AAAHC accreditation in addition to meeting AAAHC's medical home standards) or a less burdensome option called "certification" (does not require base AAAHC accreditation) (AAAHC, 2013).

c. The Joint Commission's primary care medical home designation program

The Joint Commission is an independent, not-for-profit organization, formerly known as the Joint Commission on Accreditation of Healthcare Organizations (JCAHO), which accredits and certifies nearly 21,000 healthcare organizations and programs in the United States. The Joint Commission introduced PCMH Certification for accredited ambulatory care organizations in 2011. The assessment tool is the only one based on the Agency for Healthcare Research and Quality's (AHRQ) definition of a medical home, which includes five core functions and attributes: (1) Patient-centered care; (2) Comprehensive care; (3) Coordinated care; (4) Superb access to care; (5) Systems-based approach to quality and safety (The Joint Commission, 2015a). As of December 2015, 1290 sites have received PCMH certification (The Joint Commission, 2015b).

Health Resources and Services Administration (HRSA) supports two initiatives to assist Health Center Program grantees in achieving PCMH recognition, which are the Accreditation Initiative for AAAHC and the Joint Commission program, and the Patient Centered Medical Health Home Initiative for NCQA program. According to the report from Bureau of Primary Healthcare (BPHC), 58% of federally qualified health centers (FQHC) have at least 1 site recognized as a PCMH as of October 2014.

d. Utilization Review Accreditation Committee (URAC) patient centered healthcare home program

URAC is a nonprofit organization that aims to promote healthcare quality by accrediting healthcare organizations, including health plans (HMOs, PPOs, etc.), healthcare management organizations (disease management, case management, patient-centered healthcare homes, health call centers, Independent review organizations, etc.), and health websites. URAC began offering auditor certification using their PCMH standards in 2011, which include seven core aspects: (1) Core quality care management; (2) Patient centered operations management; (3) Access and communications; (4) Testing and referrals; (5) Care management and coordination; (6) Electronic capabilities; (7) Quality performance reporting and improvement.

It's worth noting that URAC's Patient Centered Healthcare Home Program put particular emphasis on adoption of health IT, which results in applicants either being recognized for "achievement" or "achievement with electronic health records" (URAC, 2015). Table 3.1 compares the features of these national accreditation and recognition programs.

Table 3.1 Features of national accreditation and recognition programs

Organization	National Committee for Quality Assurance (NCQA)	Accreditation Association for Ambulatory Healthcare (AAAHC)	The Joint Commission	Utilization Review Accreditation Committee (URAC)
Type of the organization	An independent non-profit organization that is known for accrediting health insurance plans	A non-profit organization which accredits ambulatory healthcare organizations	An independent, not-for-profit organization, which accredits and certifies healthcare organizations and programs. Formerly known as the Joint Commission on Accreditation of Healthcare Organizations (JCAHO)	A nonprofit organization that aims to promote healthcare quality by accrediting healthcare organizations
Name of program	PCMH recognition	Medical home accreditation	Primary care medical home	Patient centered healthcare home program
Type of program	Recognition	Accreditation and certification	Accreditation and certification	Accreditation
Program begin year	2008	2009	2011	2011
Versions of standards	2008, 2011	2011, 2013	2011, 2013, 2014	2011, 2013
Core domains of the standards	Program comprises six standards: (1) Patient-centered access; (2) Team-based care; (3) Population health management; (4) Care management and support; (5) Care coordination and care transitions; (6) Performance measurement and quality improvement	Program comprises eight core standards are: (1) Patient rights and responsibilities; (2) Governance; (3) Administration; (4) Quality of care; (5) Quality management and improvement; (6) Clinical records and health information; (7) Infection prevention control and safety; (8) Facilities and environment	Program comprises five core functions and attributes: (1) Patient-centered care; (2) Comprehensive care; (3) Coordinated care; (4) Superb access to care; (5) Systems-based approach to quality and safety	Program comprises seven core aspects: (1) Core quality care management; (2) Patient centered operations management; (3) Access and communications; (4) Testing and referrals; (5) Care management and coordination; (6) Electronic capabilities; (7) Quality performance reporting and improvement

(continued)

Table 3.1 (continued)

Organization	National Committee for Quality Assurance (NCQA)	Accreditation Association for Ambulatory Healthcare (AAAHC)	The Joint Commission	Utilization Review Accreditation Committee (URAC)
Evaluation procedures	Practices complete a web-based survey tool addressing the standards for NCQA to review and verify. No mandatory site visits	Utilizes an on-site surveyor to assess applicant's performance. Applicants are required to provide supporting documentations for surveyor to review. The surveyors also conduct interviews with patients and members of the organization	Mandatory site visits are required to assess practice performance and compliance with the standards. Besides, annual basis surveys through an electronic process are required to assess practice's compliance with standards	Mandatory site visits are required. Applicants also need to provide support documentations. During the desk and on-site review process, applicants can use the web-based platform communicate with their reviewer

3.3 States' PCMH Programs

Although national accreditation or recognition standards are widely recognized, a few states—such as Minnesota and Montana—are using state level medical home standards alone or in addition to nationwide programs.

a. Minnesota's healthcare home certification program

As for the Minnesota's Healthcare Home Certification Program, it require a mandatory site visit for all applicants, and pays special attention on the quality improvement activities and health IT. Under this program, all providers are required to have an interoperable EHR by 2015. The other major categories for standards include: (1) Access/communication; (2) Patient tracking and registry functions; (3) Care coordination; (4) Care plans; (5) Performance reporting and quality improvement (Minnesota Department of Health, 2009).

b. Montana patient-centered medical home initiative

In the fall of 2009, the Montana Department of Health and Human Services began to advance a multi-payer Patient-Centered Medical Home Initiative that included Medicaid and CHIP patients. An applicant participating in the Montana PCMH program is required to obtain accreditation from one of the following nationally recognized accrediting organizations, NCQA, the Joint Commission and AAAHC. The multi-payer payment model of this imitative is designed as: Blue Cross Blue Shield of Montana pays a per member per month (PMPM) participation fee for each attributed member and a PMPM fee for chronic disease management; the two health plans (PacificSource Health Plans and Allegiance Benefit Plan Management) compensates providers with traditional FFS payments and through care coordination the Current Procedural Terminology (CPT) code; and Montana Medicaid compensates providers with traditional FFS payment and one of 3 PMPM fees for each enrolled PCMH member (Montana Department of Health and Human Services, 2015).

3.4 Other PCC Interventions and Associated Outcomes

In addition to the national and state accreditation and recognition programs, there is a multitude of PCC interventions applied in the empirical studies. As the core PCC attributes that featured in these interventions, we categorized the existing interventions into four types according to the attributes summarized above in addition to a type of combined interventions. We summarized the four types of interventions below.

a. Whole person care intervention

The attribute of PCC means that providers value a patient as a whole person; recognize and respond to the patient's complete needs. According to the existing literature, several types of interventions were designed to help patients have an ongoing relationship with a personal physician whose role is in their total care and can timely respond to the patient's complete needs. These interventions mainly focus on the contracting a personal physician, structured interviewing and consultation processes for detecting patients' health needs and concerns. For instance, Battersby et al. conducted a coordinated care trial, in which a holistic care intervention was designed by employing service coordinator and using a problem and goals (P&G) approach to identify and respond to patient's health needs and develop health plans for them. The findings from this study showed the patients in the intervention had increased utilization of community allied health services (Battersby et al., 2007). Another study applied one-hour interview to assess chronic disease patient's health needs and understanding of their own medical conditions. The results showed that the intervention were effective in producing greater patient satisfaction with the process of care (Briggs et al., 2004). Similarly, a randomized controlled trial with bipolar disorder patients showed the PCC intervention by using assessment and care planning for patients could significantly reduce the frequency of adverse event (Simon et al., 2006).

b. Patient engagement intervention

The patient engagement means that providers respect patients' needs and preferences, and that patients can obtain necessary information regarding their condition, and be able to participate in and make decisions for their own care. There is a multitude of interventions designed for improving the patient engagement. An experiment study using statement of Treatment Preferences documents for advanced care patients showed the intervention was associated with greater satisfaction with the decision-making process and less decisional conflict (Briggs et al., 2004). Another type of patient engagement is educational programs targeted to improve communication and patient involvement in care. The impact of an educational and problem-solving session was tested in a study by using a randomized controlled trial design. Compared with control group receiving usual oncology care, the intervention group receiving a nurse-led educational intervention reported higher scores for quality of life and mood (Bakitas et al., 2009). In addition to the educational intervention, the interventions targeting encouraging patients to participate in shared decision making were widely applied in many studies. The findings from such studies showed the interventions are effective in changing in patients' ways of understanding their health conditions and improving patients actively engaging in their care (Davison & Degner, 1997; Edwards et al., 2004; Krones et al., 2008; Loh et al., 2007).

c. Enhanced access intervention

Enhanced access is a one of the fundamental attributes of PCC because it is essential for helping patients overcome barriers to care, improving patient experience, patient outcomes and healthcare efficiency. Providers commit to enhancing patients' access to care by timely accommodating patient's health needs. Many interventions were implemented to reduce patient's barrier to care, including providing 24/7 access by using on-call system, after-hours and urgent care clinics, access via secure email or telephone, group visits, etc. One study using a web-based call center to arrange non-schedule visits showed intervention group have lower hospitalization rate than control group after 12 months' follow-up (Casas et al., 2006). The other study focused on Veterans Health Administration (VHA) clinic patients demonstrated that the implementation of same-day access significantly predicted fewer non-emergent and primary care treatable ED visits (Yoon et al., 2015). In term of the electronic or internet-based tools for improving visit scheduling and patient-provider communication, a study conducted in six resource-limited community clinics demonstrated that using email encounters and electronic patient portals could improve clinic efficiency and communication between patients and providers (Schickedanz et al., 2013).

d. Combined PCC intervention

In addition to the interventions with individual PCC attribute outlined above, a number of studies consisted of a number of PCC interventions together, that is, provision of an innovative or comprehensive care plan, individually tailored care, or a guided care model, etc. For example, the impact of the guided care model was tested in a cluster-randomized controlled trial at eight practices. The researchers designed the care model by integrating a registered nurse to coordinate patient's care and providing patients health education in chronic care management. Six months after baseline, the results showed the guided care improve quality of healthcare for multi-morbid older patients (Boult et al., 2008). Another study applied individually tailored care plan in addition to a self-management education session demonstrated that the integrated intervention improve patients' disease knowledge, and adherence to the treatment after 1 year of intervention (Garcia-Aymerich et al., 2007). Table 3.2 summarized main features and the related outcomes of four categories of PCC interventions implemented in the empirical studies.

3.5 The Evaluation of Patient-Centered Care

It is imperative that experience from numerous practice of PCC be captured, understood and optimized. Evaluation is essential for understanding the results of practicing PCC in various settings and for its impact on difference subgroup populations. With rigorous, comprehensive and comparable data, policy makers, providers as well as patients, will be better positioned to improve the model, achieve enhanced performance, and experience better health outcomes. This section summarizes existing evidence on the core areas of PCC measures, the options for PCC evaluation design and the appropriate data source for evaluation.

3.5.1 The Core Areas of PCC Measures

We summarized the core areas of PCC measures at multiple levels: structure, process, and outcomes. Structure describes the context in which PCC is delivered, including

Table 3.2 Summary of PCC interventions in empirical studies

Type of PCC interventions	Interventions	Outcomes
Whole person care	– Structured interview – Consultation processes – Contract personal physician whose role is in total care for patients	– Increased utilization of community allied health services (Battersby et al., 2007) – Greater satisfaction with the process of care (Briggs et al., 2004) – Reduce the frequency of adverse event (Simon et al., 2006)
Patient engagement	– Educational session targeted to improve physician–patient communication – Printed materials showing treatment options – Patient participate treatment decision making	– Greater satisfaction with the decision-making process and less decisional conflict (Briggs et al., 2004) – Higher scores for quality of life and mood (Bakitas et al., 2009) – Changes in patients' ways of understanding their health conditions and actively engaging in their care (Davison & Degner, 1997; Edwards et al., 2004; Krones et al., 2008; Loh et al., 2007)
Enhanced access	– After hours care service – 24/7 telephone or email access – Improved communication via health IT innovations	– Lower hospitalization rate (Casas et al., 2006) – Fewer non-emergent and primary care treatable ED visits (Yoon et al., 2015) – Improved clinic efficiency and overall communication between patients and providers (Schickedanz et al., 2013)
Combined interventions	– Innovative or comprehensive care plan – Individually tailored care – Guided care model	– Improved quality of healthcare for multi-morbid older persons (Boult et al., 2008) – Enhanced patients' disease knowledge, and treatment adherence after 1 year of intervention (Garcia-Aymerich et al., 2007)

financing, staff, infrastructure and equipment. At structure level, measures are widely used for assessing a practice's capabilities to get PCMH recognition or accreditation. For example, NCQA standard includes an assessment of practice's structural capabilities because evidence indicates structure and process drive outcomes. The core measures at structure level involves the implementation of incentive payment structure, the use of health IT infrastructure, and the support of team-based personnel resources, etc.

At process level, measures relate the transactions between patients and providers throughout the delivery of PCC. The core areas of PCC process measures include preventive care (e.g., the rate of receiving certain age-appropriate disease screenings, immunizations, and tests, etc.), acute care (e.g., the rate of receiving effective acute phase treatment, the referral rate, and procedures performed, etc.), and chronic disease management (e.g., health education rate, frequency of disease-specific diagnostic testing, and the enrollment rate for a specific chronic disease management program, etc.)

With respect to the outcome level, clinical outcomes, patient-reported health states, cost and utilization measures are widely used to evaluate the performance of PCC. Physiological measures, such as HbA1c values, and the control of blood pressure are commonly used to evaluate the impact of PCC on chronic disease patients; the health status, quality of life and well-being, and functional ability are also prevailing in various studies; the hospital admissions, emergency room visits, and cost-effectiveness as well as cost–benefit measures are widely presented to show the effects of PCC.

3.5.2 Evaluation Design Considerations

There were a considerable number of studies using quantitative designs to assess the impact of PCC, because many outcome measures were easily obtained from sources like claims, medical records and electronic medical records (EHRs), while the process measures were also available from various instruments and metrics to capture both patients and provider's experience of care. Besides, the quantitative study design also allows for involving a greater number of subjects to enhance the representativeness and generalization of the results, and allows for greater accuracy and objectivity of results.

In contrast, it requires more unstructured and unobtrusive method to investigate the day-to-day problems with implementing change (Curry et al., 2009). There is increasing number of studies using qualitative methods as their study design or a part of their assessment. The qualitative methods involve focus groups, and individual in-depth interviews, key informant interviews, as well as direct observation (Crabtree & Miller, 1999). The use of qualitative methods allows for capturing details and changes of the actual intervention over time, and allows for giving real-time participatory feedback to the subjects being evaluated.

An increasing collection of mixed methods strategies are also available for evaluations, in which the quantitative and qualitative components are combined (Curry et al., 2009). The quantitative and qualitative methods can be conducted sequentially or concurrently, with equal emphasis or placed different weights. For instance, a preliminary qualitative interview can be conducted to generate specific hypotheses for quantitative component or to assist the development of assessment tool for a follow-up quantitative study. This method is particularly suitable for those that include innovative PCC strategies for monitoring organizational processes and changes over time in their implementation of the new models (Stange et al., 2010). However, the methods require researcher's advanced knowledge and capabilities, as well as more intensive time and resources.

3.5.3 Main Data Source

The main potential data source for the assessment of PCC may include data from the primary source collected by the investigator and specifically designed for the testing the hypotheses, it may also involves secondary data, such as medical record/EHR, administrative databases (such as Medicare and Medicaid claims), encounter-level databases (such as various nationally representative surveys), and medical chart abstraction, etc. The determination on types of data being used is not only based on the research aims and hypotheses, but also depends on the resources available and research time frame.

References

Accreditation Association for Ambulatory Health Care. (2013). *Accreditation association for ambulatory health care.* Accessed on January 8, 2016. Available at: http://www.nhchc.org/wp-content/uploads/2014/12/whats-in-our-medical-home.pdf.

Accreditation Association for Ambulatory Health Care. (2015). *Medical home accreditation.* Accessed on January 8, 2016. Available at: http://www.aaahc.org/accreditation/primary-care-medical-home/.

Agency for Healthcare Research and Quality. (2015). *PCMH Foundations.* Accessed on January 8, 2016. Available at: https://pcmh.ahrq.gov/page/pcmh-foundations.

Bakitas, M., Lyons, K. D., Hegel, M. T., Balan, S., Brokaw, F. C., Seville, J., Hull, J. G., Li, Z., Tosteson, T. D., Byock, I. R., & Ahles, T. A. (2009). Effects of a palliative care intervention on clinical outcomes in patients with advanced cancer: The Project ENABLE II randomized controlled trial. *JAMA, 302*(7), 741–749.

Bates, D. W., & Bitton, A. (2010). The future of health information technology in the patient-centered medical home. *Health Affairs (millwood), 29*(4), 614–621.

Battersby, M., Harvey, P., Mills, P. D., Kalucy, E., Pols, R. G., Frith, P. A., McDonald, P., Esterman, A., Tsourtos, G., Donato, R., Pearce, R., & McGowan, C. (2007). SA HealthPlus: A controlled trial of a statewide application of a generic model of chronic illness care. *Milbank Quarterly, 85*(1), 37–67.

Bodenheimer, T., Wagner, E. H., & Grumbach, K. (2002). Improving primary care for patients with chronic illness: The chronic care model, Part 2. *JAMA, 288*(15), 1909–1914.

Bojadzievski, T., & Gabbay, R. A. (2011). Patient-centered medical home and diabetes. *Diabetes Care, 34*(4), 1047–1053.

Boult, C., Karm, L., & Groves, C. (2008). Improving chronic care: The "guided care" model. *The Permanente Journal, 12*(1), 50–54.

Briggs, L. A., Kirchhoff, K. T., Hammes, B. J., Song, M. K., & Colvin, E. R. (2004). Patient-centered advance care planning in special patient populations: A pilot study. *Journal of Professional Nursing, 20*(1), 47–58.

Casas, A., Troosters, T., Garcia-Aymerich, J., Roca, J., Hernandez, C., Alonso, A., del Pozo, F., de Toledo, P., Anto, J. M., Rodriguez-Roisin, R., & Decramer, M. (2006). Integrated care prevents hospitalisations for exacerbations in COPD patients. *European Respiratory Journal, 28*(1), 123–130.

Centers for Medicare and Medicaid Services. (2015). *FQHC advanced primary care practice demonstration*. Accessed on January 8, 2016. Available at: https://innovation.cms.gov/initiatives/fqhcs/.

Coleman, K., Austin, B. T., Brach, C., & Wagner, E. H. (2009). Evidence on the Chronic Care Model in the new millennium. *Health Affairs (millwood), 28*(1), 75–85.

Crabtree, B. F., & Miller, W. L. (1999). *Doing qualitative research*. Sage Publications.

Curry, L. A., Nembhard, I. M., & Bradley, E. H. (2009). Qualitative and mixed methods provide unique contributions to outcomes research. *Circulation, 119*(10), 1442–1452.

Davison, B. J., & Degner, L. F. (1997). Empowerment of men newly diagnosed with prostate cancer. *Cancer Nursing, 20*(3), 187–196.

Department of Health and Human Services. (2012). *Fact sheet: Medicare-medicaid advanced primary care demonstration initiative*. Accessed on January 8, 2016. Available at: https://innovation.cms.gov/Files/fact-sheet/mapcpdemo-Fact-Sheet.pdf.

Edwards, A., Elwyn, G., Hood, K., Atwell, C., Robling, M., Houston, H., Kinnersley, P., Russell, I., & G. Study Steering. (2004). Patient-based outcome results from a cluster randomized trial of shared decision making skill development and use of risk communication aids in general practice. *Family Practice, 21*(4), 347–354.

Garcia-Aymerich, J., Hernandez, C., Alonso, A., Casas, A., Rodriguez-Roisin, R., Anto, J. M., & Roca, J. (2007). Effects of an integrated care intervention on risk factors of COPD readmission. *Respiratory Medicine, 101*(7), 1462–1469

Kongstvedt, P. R. (2007). *Essentials of managed health care*. Jones and Bartlett.

Krones, T., Keller, H., Sonnichsen, A., et al. (2008). Absolute cardiovascular disease risk and shared decision making in primary care: A randomized controlled trial. *Annals of Family Medicine, 6*, 218–227.

Loh, A., Simon, D., Wills, C. E., Kriston, L., Niebling, W., & Harter, M. (2007). The effects of a shared decision-making intervention in primary care of depression: A cluster-randomized controlled trial. *Patient Education and Counseling, 67*(3), 324–332.

Maeng, D. D., Khan, N., Tomcavage, J., Graf, T. R., Davis, D. E., & Steele, G. D. (2015). Reduced acute inpatient care was largest savings component of Geisinger Health System's patient-centered medical home. *Health Affairs (millwood), 34*(4), 636–644.

Minnesota Department of Health. (2009). *An overview of health care homes in Minnesota*. Accessed on January 8, 2016. Available at: http://www.health.state.mn.us/healthreform/homes/about/HCH_FactSheet.pdf.

Montana Department of Health and Human Services. (2015). *Montana patient centered medical home program 2015 public report*. Accessed on January 8, 2016. Available at: http://csimt.gov/wp-content/uploads/2015PCMHPublicReport_Final.pdf.

National Committee for Quality Assurance (NCQA). (2008). *Standards and guidelines for physician practice connections—patient-centered medical home*. Accessed on January 8, 2016. Available at: http://www.ncqa.org/Portals/0/Programs/Recognition/PCMH_Overview_Apr01.pdf.

National Committee for Quality Assurance (NCQA). (2014). *The future of patient-centered medical homes: foundation for a better health care system*. Accessed on January 8, 2016. Available at:http://www.ncqa.org/Portals/0/Public%20Policy/2014%20Comment%20Letters/The_Future_of_PCMH.pdf.

Paulus, R. A., Davis, K., & Steele, G. D. (2008). Continuous innovation in health care: Implications of the Geisinger experience. *Health Affairs (millwood), 27*(5), 1235–1245.

Schickedanz, A., Huang, D., Lopez, A., Cheung, E., Lyles, C. R., Bodenheimer, T., & Sarkar, U. (2013). Access, interest, and attitudes toward electronic communication for health care among patients in the medical safety net. *Journal of General Internal Medicine, 28*(7), 914–920.

Simon, G. E., Ludman, E. J., Bauer, M. S., Unutzer, J., & Operskalski, B. (2006). Long-term effectiveness and cost of a systematic care program for bipolar disorder. *Archives of General Psychiatry, 63*(5), 500–508.

Stange, K. C., Nutting, P. A., Miller, W. L., Jaen, C. R., Crabtree, B. F., Flocke, S. A., & Gill, J. M. (2010). Defining and measuring the patient-centered medical home. *Journal of General Internal Medicine, 25*(6), 601–612.

The Joint Commission. (2015a). *Facts about primary care medical home certification*. Accessed on January 8, 2016. Available at: http://www.jointcommission.org/facts_about_primary_care_medical_home_certification/.

The Joint Commission. (2015b). *Joint commission accredited organizations with Primary Care Medical Home (PCMH) Certification*. Accessed on January 8, 2016. Available at: http://www.jointcommission.org/assets/1/18/PCMH_org_list.pdf.

Utilization Review Accreditation Committee (URAC). (2015). *Patient centered health care home program*. Accessed on January 8, 2016. Available at: https://www.urac.org/accreditation-and-measurement/accreditation-programs/all-programs/patient-centered-medical-home/.

Wagner, E. H., Austin, B. T., & Von Korff, M. (1996). Organizing care for patients with chronic illness. *Milbank Quarterly, 74*(4), 511–544.

Wagner, E. H., Austin, B. T., & Von Korff, M. (1996). Improving outcomes in chronic illness. *Managed Care Quarterly, 4*(2), 12–25.

Wagner, E. H., Davis, C., Schaefer, J., Von Korff, M., & Austin, B. (1999). A survey of leading chronic disease management programs: Are they consistent with the literature? *Managed Care Quarterly, 7*(3), 56–66.

Wagner, E. H., Glasgow, R. E., Davis, C., Bonomi, A. E., Provost, L., McCulloch, D., Carver, P., & Sixta, C. (2001). Quality improvement in chronic illness care: A collaborative approach. *Joint Commission Journal on Quality Improvement, 27*(2), 63–80.

Yoon, J., Cordasco, K. M., Chow, A., & Rubenstein, L. V. (2015). The relationship between same-day access and continuity in primary care and emergency department visits. *PLoS One, 10*(9), e0135274.

Chapter 4
Patient-Centered Care and Elderly Healthcare

4.1 Patient-Centered Care on Older Adults with Chronic Conditions

Due to the dynamic health status and the use of multiple types of healthcare providers, delivering care to older patients with chronic conditions is challenging. On one hand, treatments for older adults with chronic conditions are complicated, especially when patients with multiple chronic conditions. In some circumstances, treatments improve one outcome may worsen outcome. For example, it is known that many of the medications used to treat heart failure may worsen kidney function. At the same time, healthcare providers may also need to fear the liability regarding both unnecessary interventions and underuse of therapies. On the other hand, it's very difficult to explain the benefits and harms to the patients when physicians need to make multiple simultaneous decisions and treatment, which make patients and their families hard to get active involvement in decisions making (Wolff et al., 2009). To overcome these challenges, numerous studies and policies are trying to promote paradigm shift from the traditional provider-driven care model to patient actively engaged care model, and highlighted the patient's role in their own chronic disease management.

The ACA provides new opportunities for PCC to manage chronic conditions through designing and piloting of new types of PCC to coordinate care and therefore enhance the quality of care and patients' benefits. Specifically, a new Center for Medicare and Medicaid Innovation are developed to examine approaches to health coordination and improvement. From the states level, health homes for Medicaid enrollees are providing to patients with chronic conditions. All of those efforts are connected to Healthy People 2020, which is served as the basis of is the national health objectives as well as the development of local healthcare plans.

Now is the time to view the impact of PCC on chronic disease prevention and care management. Better evidence on methods and outcomes of the model is needed to enhance the care provided for older adults with chronic conditions. However, according to the existing literature, it was difficult to draw firm conclusions regarding

H. Liang, *The Impact of Patient-Centered Care*,
https://doi.org/10.1007/978-981-16-3968-5_4

the best PCC approaches for managing chronic conditions among older adults. Most interventions in the current literature included PCC as attempts to educate patients or get them involved into the whole process of treatment decision making. Other common approaches related on training health providers in delivering empowering PCC. One study conducted by Wagner et al. (2012) found that empowering patients by increasing their capacity to engage with providers is related to patient-reported improvements in the quality of care, but not in patient satisfaction. The study conducted by Sullivan et al. (2006) suggested that providers who received PCC training were more likely to report positive relationships with patients and agreement about care. However, the best approaches of PCC applied for older adults with chronic conditons remain unclear. There is also very little knowledge on the most improtant attributes required for PCC delivery and whether it enhances patient perceived satisfaction, health outcomes, safety, and efficiency. In addition, there was no nationwide evidence to our knowledge that particularly focused on the benefits of PCC for older adults with chornic conditions. Therefore, our study is designed to fill this specific knowledge gaps.

4.2 Conceptual Framework for Evluation

The conceptual framework of this evaluation (Fig. 4.1) is adapted from Donabedian's structure, process, and outcome model (Donabedian, 1966). Donabedian's framework is one of the most widely used models for assessment of quality in the healthcare services field. According to this framework, it classified inferences about the quality of care into three categories: structure, process and outcome. The part of structure includes the attributes of the healthcare settings in which care occurs, which encompasses organizational structure, facilities, equipment, financial and human resources. The process includes the activities in providing and receiving healthcare. In this study,

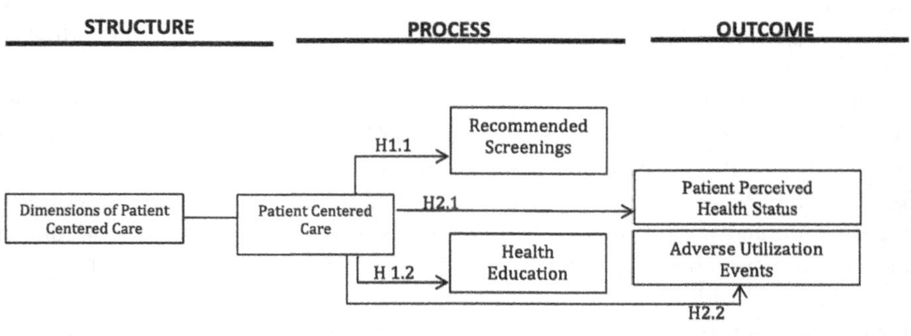

Fig. 4.1 Conceptual framework of the study. *Source* Donabedian (1988)

we propose to assess the relationship between PCC and measures of chronic management among older adults, including receipt of preventive screening and health education for chronic diseases. The outcome dimension includes the impact of healthcare on patients' health status. In this study, we propose to assess the relationship between PCC and chronic disease health outcomes, including patient perceived health status and incidence of adverse utilization events.

4.3 Study Aims and Research Questions

4.3.1 Study Objectives

The objective of the empirical sections are to investigate the impact of PCC for older adults with chronic conditions, and to add evidence of its effects on patient's experiences, process of care, and health outcomes.

4.3.2 Specific Aims

The following chapters are designed to address two specific aims as follows. These aims are inter-related, focusing the objective of the study, that is, to reveal the heterogeneous nature of PCC, prioritize guided efforts for a sustainable development of PCC in chronic condition management for older adults and explore factors that shape the impact of PCC. In our study, we define older adults as adults aged 65 years or older according to the guideline from the Centers for Disease Control and Prevention (Centers for Disease Control and Prevention, 2013b).

Specific Aim 1: To assess the association between the receipt of PCC and chronic management among older adults, measured by the receipt of preventive screening and health education for chronic diseases.

Specific Aim 2: To assess the association between the receipt of PCC and chronic disease health outcomes among older adults, measured by patient perceived health status and incidence of adverse utilization events.

PCC initiatives are central to many efforts to reform the US healthcare delivery system. Although some studies show promise regarding the benefits of PCC, it still requires additional study to show if PCC is applicable to a specific patient population demanding complex healthcare needs. That's why we chose older adults with chronic conditions as our target population.

Under the legislation highlighting the importance of patient-centered outcomes research in the ACA, there is increased attention in both research and clinical sectors. It need nation-wide representative data to investigate the current impact of PCC.

4.3.3 Hypotheses

Specific Aim 1: Hypothesis 1.1: Thre receipt of PCC is associated with increased preventive screenings delivered to older adults with chronic conditions.

Hypothesis 1.2: Thre receipt of PCC is associated with increased health education provided to older adults with chronic conditions.

Specific Aim 2: Hypothesis 2.1: Thre receipt of PCC is associated with good patient perceived health status.

Hypothesis 2.2: Thre receipt of PCC is associated with fewer adverse healthcare utilization events.

4.4 Data and Sample

4.4.1 Medical Expenditure Panel Survey

The data for this study came from the Medical Expenditure Panel Survey (MEPS), a nationally representative 2-year panel survey of non-institutionalized, US civilian families and individuals, administrative by the AHRQ. There are three components of MEPS: the Household Component, the Medical Provider component and the Insurance/Employer Component. The Household Component (HC) draws the sampling frame from a nationally representative subsample of National Health Interview Survey (NHIS), which is conducted by the National Center for Health Statistics. The NHIS is a complex multi-stage sample design, which consist two stages. The first stage of sample selection is an area sample of Primary Sampling Units (PSUs), where PSUs generally consist of one or more counties. The second-stage of sample selection includes area segments within a PSU, consisting of clusters of housing units, and also reflecting the density of minority populations. Since 2006, Asians are oversampled in addition to Blacks and Hispanics. Sample weights are used to adjust the disproportionate contribution from oversampled subgroups (Ezzati-Rice et al., 2008).

By using computer assisted personal interviewing (CAPI) technology, all data for a sampled household are reported by one designated household respondent. In general, the reference person is identified as the household member 16 years of age or older who owns or rents the home. As a complex national probability survey, the MEPS-HC was initiated in 1996. By using the overlapping panel design of the survey, data are collected through a series of five rounds of interviews covering 2 full calendar years. Each year a new panel of sample households is selected, that means data are collected simultaneously for two panels during each calendar year. As illustrated in Table 4.1, one panel is in its first year of interviews (e.g., in the year 2013, Rounds 1, 2, and 3 of Panel 18), while the prior year's panel is in its second year of data collection (e.g., in 2013, Rounds 3, 4, and 5 of Panel 17) (Cohen et al., 1997). AHRQ rearranges the data into yearly files, which provide summarized

Table 4.1 Sample frames by year and by panel, MEPS 2009–2013

	Panel	Year	Sample Size	Year Total	Panel Total
2013	18	1	18,092	36,940	18,092
	17	2	18,848		38,562
2012	17	1	19,714	38,974	
	16	2	19,260		39,357
2011	16	1	20,097	35,313	
	15	2	15,216		31,068
2010	15	1	15,852	32,846	
	14	2	16,994		34,638
2009	14	1	17,644	36,855	
	13	2	19,211		19,211
Total				180,928	180,928

Source MEPS Consolidated File Documentation, 2009–2013

information for 1-year observation periods. In most years, the MEPS-HC samples are not completely independent because each MEPS respondent can contribute up to two person-year observations. The variable DUPERSID in the dataset can be used as an identifier to indicate that the 2 observations came from a same person. However, DUPERSID uniquely identifies a MEPS sample person only within a full-year data file containing adjacent panels. As we were pooling multiple years of data, we used a combination of DUPERSID and PANEL as the identifier because some DUPERSID values have been used in multiple panels. We used 1:1 match merge to identify and correct duplicate identifiers.

The target population in this study is older adults aged 65 and beyond with at least one chronic condition. To yield sample sizes to generate reliable estimates, it is desirable to pool together multiple data to facilitate analysis. Although MEPS-HC samples are not completely independent because many people are in the sample for two consecutive years and the households being interviewed are selected from the same geographic areas, it is still valid to pool more than one year of data. It is because that each year of the MEPS-HC is designed to be nationally representative, and the annual data files are released with one common variance structure, which reflects the complex sample design of the MEPS-HC and can be used for pooling the data (AHRQ, 2009).

4.4.2 Sample Size and Power

The Full-Year Consolidated MEPS-HC Data Files 2009 through 2013 provided the data source for this study. Table 4.1 provides the sampling frame for MEPS-HC for the 2009–2013 year period. Response rates for the MEPS-HC full-year data from

2009 to 2013 ranged from 52.8 to 57.2%, which reflects nonresponse to the NHIS from which the MEPS-HC is drawn, as well as the nonresponse and attrition in MEPS-HC.

To maintain the integrity of the MEPS survey design, we kept all the records from all the respondents accounted for by the full set of survey stratum and PSU values. We generated a flag variable for all survey respondents that were used to identify our target samples, rather than creating a sub-file that contain only respondents in the subdomain of interest. MEPS-HC contains variables pertaining to survey administration, demographics, income, person-level conditions, health status, disability days, quality of care, employment, health insurance, and person-level medical care use and expenditures (Cohen et al., 2009), from which we can collects high-quality information describing chronic care services and variables essential for examining the patient-centered care as well as healthcare performance.

Patients are the unit of analysis for all specific aims. To estimate the power for our analyses, we use a dataset with 16,654 patient (the total sample size of the pooled data is 180,928, we included sample aged older than 65, having at least one chronic condition, and having usual source of care; we excluded samples with duplicates identifiers, missing or ineligible value on independent and/or variables). Figure 4.2 provides the details of creating the analytic samples and the numbers of included respondents for each outcome variable of this study. Based on an estimated 9 percent difference in the delivery of a cholesterol screening service with a standard deviation of 5 between patient with and without PCC (Beal et al., 2009), the power of the analysis is estimated above the recommended minimum of 80% (Ellis, 2010).

4.4.3 Strategies for Addressing Missing Values

We treated missing value based on the assessment of data quality in terms of number, percentage, mean and percentage of missing data. The proportion of missing for independent variables and covariates were small (less than 5% in total). Based on the inference that item-missing rates less than 5% are not likely to produce major biases for survey estimates based on only the complete cases (Heeringa et al., 2010), and using substitution method were considered to be acceptable (Dong & Peng, 2013; Little & Rubin, 1989; Rubin, 1998), we did not use multiple imputations for imputing the missing independent variables and covariates. And we substituted the missing values for three covariates (employment status, ADLs, and IADLs) using previous panel rounds of the same variable to complete the missing values. For the rest of missing covariates and independent variables that have no previous panel rounds values to substitute, we exclude these respondents with missing values. In summary, the total substation and drops due to missing values of covariates and independent variables were 4.44%. For the dependent variables, we conducted complete case analyses rather than imputation. The final sample size for the each dependent variable is showed in Fig. 4.1. Besides the rational above, to inform these decisions about imputation and drops, we also performed sensitivity analyses (van Houwelingen et al.,

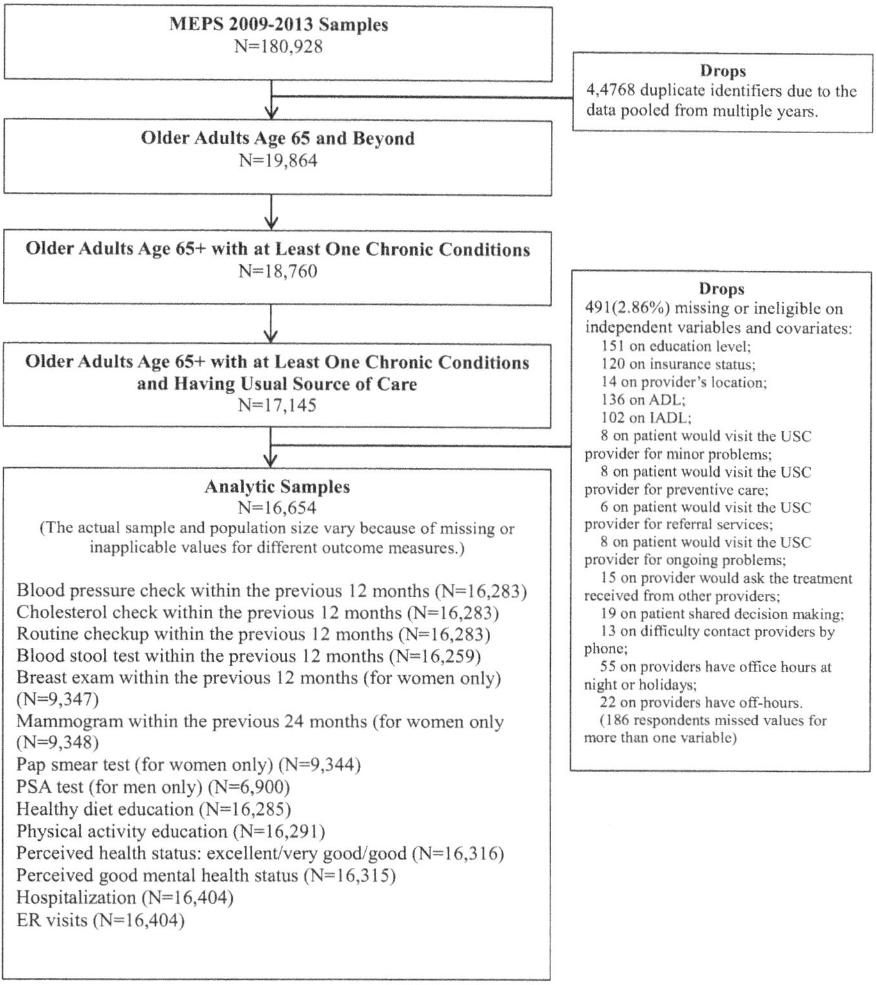

Fig. 4.2 Analytic samples

2011). Excluded respondents were compared to the analytic sample. The analysis was weighted to account for the complex survey design by using the svy commands available in Stata. Table 4.2 presents the results of the sensitivity analysis and shows that the excluded individuals are not systematically different from those included in SES status (Adler, 1994) and PCC status, which further shows that conducting complete case analyses are appropriate.

Table 4.2 Sensitivity analyses: weighted analytic samples compared to excluded samples

	Analytic sample	Excluded sample
Sample size (unweighted)	16,654	491
Weighted population (1000)	181,599.05	4,498.96
Age	74.28	74.87
Number of chronic conditions*	3.91	3.76
Socioeconomic status		
Education (%)		
No degree	19.58	22.36
General equivalency diploma/high school diploma	42.68	41.29
Bachelor's degree/some college/associate degree	21.86	21.01
Advance degree	15.88	15.34
Employment status (%)		
Not employed	80.91	83.01
Employed	19.09	16.99
Household per capita income (Mean, SE)*	311,10.42	298,12.68
PCC Status (%)		
PCC	35.65	34.59
Partial PCC	41.94	39.60
Non-PCC	22.40	25.81

*$P < 0.05$, results based on t test continuous measures and design-based F test for categorical measures

4.5 Measures

For this study, we used measures of PCC attributes (independent variables), chronic condition management/patient perceived health status/adverse events (dependent variables), and individual characteristics (covariates) that have potentially confounding effects on the experience of PCC.

4.5.1 Independent Variables

A majority of the previous literature derived PCC measures based on structural and process measures reported by healthcare providers or based on recognition records from health administrative agencies. However, patient reports of their experiences with care are being used more and more to develop robust indicators of PCC (Beal et al., 2009; Schoen et al., 2007). In accordance with the synthesized attributes in Chap. 2, the previous literature (Beal et al., 2009) and the results from the exploratory factor analysis (EFA), we operationalize three distinctive attributes of PCC—whole person care, patient engagement, and enhanced access of care. The process of extracting PCC attributes is described as follows.

Using MEPS-HC data, we initially selected nine items to measuring the PCC.

These items selection was based on the synthesized attributes in Chap. 2 and a previous study (Beal et al., 2009). The nine variables used for measuring PCC attributes were selected from the items in the Access to Care (AC) section of the MEPS HC questionnaire. There was no specific time period referred to for these items in the questionnaire. We consider the time period is the past 12 months, based on the other questions referred to in this AC section. Table 4.3 shows the original questionnaire questions and answer options, percentage of missing and other details of these items in MEPS.

In our study, the EFA was used to explore the structure of PCC measures and examine their construct. The EFA is a variable reduction technique which identifies the factors account for common variance in the data, and estimates factors underlying construct that cannot be measured directly (Suhr, 2005). We used the EFA to explore the possible underlying factor structure of PCC by a set of measured variables in the MEPS. The standard methods of factor analysis assume that the measurement scale is interval of ratio level follow a normal distribution. If the model includes variables that are dichotomous a factor analysis can be conducted using a tetrachoric or polychoric correlation matrix (UCLA Statistical Consulting Group, 2015). In Stata we first generate a matrix of tetrachoric correlations by using a user-written command tetrachoric. Then we perform the EFA and determine number of factors to retain. Factor loadings are considered significant if they are 0.40 or higher (Fayers & Hand, 1997). Due to the nature of survey data in this study, the results are based on the exploratory factor analysis using the tetrachoric correlation as input, rather than raw variables (van der Eijk & Rose, 2015). Table 4.4 shows the results of factor analysis, which verifies the three common factors extracted from nine items.

USC: usual source of care

According to the results from the EFA, we extracted three factors underlying the construct of PCC.

(1) Whole person care: Four different facets of the person's level of confidence in the usual source of care (USC) provider are examined: Is the provider the person or place family members would go to for routine or minor health problems (MINORP42), preventive healthcare (PREVEN42), referrals to other health professionals (REFFRL42), and ongoing health problems (ONGONG42).
(2) Patient engagement in care: USC provider always or usually ask about prescription medications and treatments other doctors may give them (TREATM42), or ask the person to help make decisions between a choice of treatments (DECIDE42)
(3) Enhanced care accessibility: the respondent has no difficulty of accessing the USC provider by phone (PHNREG42), the USC provider has office hours at night or on the weekend (OFFHOU42), or the respondent has no difficulty of accessing the USC provider after hours (AFTHOU42).

Table 4.3 MEPS items used for measuring patient-centered care attributes

Variable	Items and answer options	N (%) of missing	Variable value = 1 N (%)
Confidence in USC for routine or minor health problems (MINORP42)	Is the USC provider you and your family members would go to for routine or new minor health problems? (Yes vs. No)	8 (0.05)	16,399 (98.46)
Confidence in USC for preventive healthcare (PREVEN42)	Is the USC provider you and your family members would go to for preventive healthcare? (Yes vs. No)	8 (0.05)	16,403 (98.49)
Confidence in USC for ongoing health problems (ONGONG42)	Is the USC provider you and your family members would go to for referrals to other health professionals? (Yes vs. No)	6 (0.03)	16,316 (97.97)
Confidence in USC for referrals to other health professionals (REFFRL42)	Is the USC provider you and your family members would go to for ongoing health problems? (Yes vs. No)	8 (0.05)	16,275 (97.72)
Usually ask about prescription medications and treatments other doctors may give them (TREATM42)	Does your USC provider usually ask about prescription medications and treatments other doctors may give them? (Yes vs. No)	15 (0.09)	13,011 (78.13)
Always or usually ask the person to help make decisions between a choice of treatments (DECIDE42)	If there were a choice between treatments, how often would your USC provider ask you to help make the decision? (Always/usually vs. Sometime/never)	19 (0.11)	12,773 (76.70)
Has no difficulty of accessing the USC provider by phone (PHNREG42)	How difficult is it to contact your USC provider during regular business hours over the telephone about a health problem? (Not at all/not too difficult vs. somewhat/very difficult)	13 (0.08)	13,496 (81.04)
USC provider has office hours at night or on the weekend (OFFHOU42)	Does your USC provider have office hours at night or on weekends? (Yes vs. No)	55 (0.32)	4,253 (25.54)

(continued)

Table 4.3 (continued)

Variable	Items and answer options	N (%) of missing	Variable value = 1 N (%)
Has no difficulty of accessing the USC provider after hours (AFTHOU42)	How difficult is it to contact your USC provider after their regular hours in case of urgent medical needs? (Not at all/not too difficult vs. somewhat/very difficult)	22 (0.12)	6,805 (40.86)

Table 4.4 Factor loading of patient-centered care measures

	Whole person care	Patient engagement	Enhanced accessibility
Confidence in USC for routine or minor health problems	0.49	0.02	0.05
Confidence in USC for preventive healthcare	0.51	0.001	–0.06
Confidence in USC for ongoing health problems	0.49	0.03	–0.01
Confidence in USC for referrals to other health professionals	0.50	–0.05	0.01
Usually ask about prescription medications and treatments other doctors may give them	-0.02	0.65	0.02
Always or usually ask the person to help make decisions between a choice of treatments	0.02	0.61	0.15
Has no difficulty of accessing the USC provider by phone	0.05	0.23	0.47
USC provider has office hours at night or on the weekend	0.01	–0.38	0.59
Has no difficulty of accessing the USC provider after hours	–0.05	0.12	0.64

USC: usual source of care.

Table 4.5 Patient-centered care status and samples

	Freq	Percent	Cum. Percent
PCC	5963	35.81	35.81
Partial PCC	6973	41.87	77.68
Non-PCC	3718	22.32	100
Total	16,654	100	

Using the items listed above, respondents were categorized into three groups: (1) having PCC (those who said yes to all items in the whole person care domain, has at least one yes in each patient engagement domain and enhanced accessibility domain, and said yes to at least 8 items in total); (2) having partial PCC (those who said yes to all items in the whole person care domain, has at least one yes in each patient engagement domain and enhanced accessibility domain); (3) Non-PCC (those who said no to any item in the whole person care domain, or has no item in patient engagement domain and/or enhanced accessibility domain). Based on this method, the total included samples were categorized into three groups. Table 4.5 shows the samples size in the each group.

As we would also perform multivariate logistic regression on the associating PCC attributes with the each outcome variables. We defined the each attribute of PCC as follows. (1) "whole person care versus non-whole person care": patients who said yes to all four items in the whole person care domain are defined as having "whole person care"; (2) "patient engagement versus non-patient engagement": patients who said yes to both items in the patient engagement domain are defined as having "patient engagement"; and (3) "enhanced access versus non-enhanced access": patients who said yes to all three items in the enhanced access domain are defined as having "enhanced access".

4.5.2 Dependent Variables

The dependent variables include variables regarding chronic condition management measured by the receipt of preventive screenings and the receipt of health education, and the health outcome variables measured by patient perceived health status and adverse utilization events.

(1) Receipt of Recommended Screenings: We measured the receipt of eight types of screenings, which are: blood pressure check within the past year, blood cholesterol check within the past year, routine check-up within the past year, blood stool test within the past year, breast exam within the past year (for female only), mammogram check within the past 2 year (for female only), ever have a Pap smear test (for women only), and ever have a prostate specific antigen test (for male only). For each specific screening, we adjust for age and risk, according to the Guide to Clinical Preventive Services includes U.S. Preventive

Table 4.6 Description and inclusion criteria for each screening measure

Variable name in MEPS	Screening measures	Coding method	Inclusion criteria
CHECK53	Blood pressure	1 Yes, 2 No	Patients aged $\geq$ 65 years
CHOLCK53	Blood cholesterol	1 Yes, 2 No	Patients aged $\geq$ 65 years
BPCHEK53	Routine check-up	1 Yes, 2 No	Patients aged $\geq$ 65 years
BSTST53	Blood stool test	1 Yes, 2 No	Patients aged $\geq$ 65 years
BRSTEX53	Breast exam	1 Yes, 2 No	Female patients aged $\geq$ 65 years
MAMOGR53	Mammography	1 Yes, 2 No	Female patients aged $\geq$ 65 years
PAPSMR53	Pap smear test	1 Yes, 2 No	Female patients aged $\geq$ 65 years
PSA53	Prostate specific antigen	1 Yes, 2 No	Men aged $\geq$ 65 years

Services Task Force (USPSTF) recommendations on screening, counseling, and preventive medication. It should be noted that the USPSTF recommends against prostate-specific antigen (PSA)-based screening for prostate cancer due to the high over-diagnosis rate according to the latest 2015 guideline. However, based on the guideline update in 2001, the PSA test should be offered annually, beginning at age 50, to men who have a life expectancy of at least 10 years, and to younger men who are at high risk. Due to part of the MEPS data were collected before the new guideline updates, we still use the previous guideline for evaluating the receipt of preventive services. The finalized variables derived from survey items representing each measure can be found in Table 4.6.

(2) Receipt of Health Education: We measured the receipt of two types of health education within the past year: advice on more exercise (EXRCIS53), and advice on healthy diet (NOFAT53). We coded these variables into dichotomous variables in Yes versus No.
(3) Patient Perceived Health Status: We assessed patient perceived physical health status (ADGENH42) and mental health status (PHQ242). We coded these variables into dichotomous variables in excellent/very good/good versus fair/poor.
(4) Adverse Utilization: adverse utilization in the past year that may reflect poor chronic conditions control. We measured the number of emergency department (ED) visits (ERTOT) and the happening of hospitalizations event (IPDIS). We coded the ER visits and happening of hospitalizations event into dichotomous variables in Yes versus No.

4.5.3 Covariates

We use the Aday and Andersen's access framework (Aday et al., 1984) to select covariates that are related to the experience of patient-centered care. The framework was designed to identify both individual and contextual determinants of medical care utilization. According to the model, the utilization of health services is determined by three dynamics: predisposing factors, enabling factors, and need factors. The original model was developed by in 1968, and was expanded through numerous iterations (Andersen, 1995). The Aday and Andersen's access framework has been applied extensively to guide the health services research design and to predict health care utilization behaviors.

By using this framework, we identified individual and system factors that influenced the healthcare use. Specifically, individual factors include predisposing, enabling, and need. Predisposing factors are biologically or socially constructed factors that influence individual's inclination to use healthcare services, such as age, gender, racial and ethnic identity, education level, and health belief factors, etc. Enabling factors are the resources and the ability of an individual and availability of healthcare services that enable the use of healthcare. These factors may include income, health insurance status, ability to travel, and distance to a healthcare provider, etc. Need factors are the individual's objective and subjective needs for healthcare services. These factors may include existing health conditions, symptoms, disabilities, and self or socially evaluated health needs, etc. System factors typically include factors regarding policies, organization, financing that influence healthcare services delivery (Phillips et al., 1998). Based on the model, we selected covariates for this study. These measures as well as their coding are shown in Table 4.7. We did not include a time variable to control for trends over time, because we initially performed bivariate analyses and the results showed that the 14 outcome measures did not change over five years from 2009 to 2013, and our study's primary hypotheses were not regarding to the time change. Table 4.8 showed each of the 14 dependent variables over the years from 2009 to 2013.

4.6 Sample Weights and Variance Structure

The design of the MEPS includes clustering, multiple stages and disproportionate sampling. Additionally, the nonresponse was adjusted by using sampling weights. Therefore, special considerations on the survey design were required. In order to obtain correct estimates and accurate standard error for either descriptive statistics or multivariate models, the survey design complexities need to be taken into account by using an appropriate technique to derive accurate weighted estimates (Machlin et al., 2005). Therefore, all the analyses in this study were weighted to reflect the complex

Table 4.7 Description for each covariate

	Description	Coding method	% of missing
Predisposing factors	Age	Continuous	0
	Gender	Male versus female	0
	Race/ethnicity	1. Non-Hispanic white, 2. Hispanic, 3. Black, 4. Non-Hispanic Asian, 5. Non-Hispanic other race or multi-races	0
	Marriage	Married versus not married	0
	Highest education	1. No degree, 2. general equivalency diploma/high school diploma, 3. Bachelor's degree/some college/associate degree, 4. advance degree	151 (0.88)
	Employment status	Employed versus not employed	
	Census region	1. Northeast, 2. Midwest, 3. South, 4. West	0
Enabling factors	Household per capita income	Continuous	0
	Insurance coverage	1. Uninsured, 2. Medicare only, 3. Medicare and private, 4. Medicare and other public only, 5. no Medicare and any public/private	120 (0.70)
Need factors	Need help with activities of daily living (ADLs)	Yes versus No	136 (0.79)
	Need Help with Instrumental Activities of Daily Living (IADLs)	Yes versus No	102 (0.59)
	Number of chronic conditions	Continuous	0
	Provider's types	1. Person, 2. Facility, 3. Person in facility provider	0
	Provider's Location	1. Office, 2. Hospital, not ER, 3. Hospital, ER	14 (0.08)

survey design of MEPS. We used the variables: primary sampling unit (PSU), person-level estimation weight (p weight) and sampling strata (varstr) variables in the MEPS to obtain weighted estimates.

Table 4.8 Weighted dependent variables by year, 2009–2013

	Total	2009	2010	2011	2012	2013	*P* Value
Sample size (unweighted)	16,654	3197	3050	3421	3607	3379	–
Weighted population (1000)	181,599.05	33,157.26	33,861.63	36,216.69	37,777.59	39,383.89	–
Blood pressure check within the previous 12 months (N = 16,283)	97.57	97.63	97.40	97.37	97.58	97.84	0.81
Cholesterol check within the previous 12 months (N = 16,283)	91.66	90.33	91.57	91.81	92.27	92.14	0.23
Routine checkup within the previous 12 months (N = 16,283)	91.11	90.45	90.68	92.05	91.27	91.01	0.45
Blood stool test within the previous 12 months (N = 16,259)	18.81	20.87	19.83	20.20	16.11	17.52	0.11
Breast exam within the previous 12 months (only for women) (N = 9347)	59.61	60.04	59.29	59.67	58.62	60.44	0.87
Mammogram within the previous 24 months (only for women) (N = 9348)	73.55	72.93	75.35	74.30	72.82	72.52	0.36
Pap smear test (only for women) (N = 9344)	95.99	95.73	96.23	95.50	96.28	96.17	0.79
PSA test (only for men) (N = 6900)	68.65	71.35	69.76	68.13	68.02	66.62	0.19

(continued)

Table 4.8 (continued)

	Total	2009	2010	2011	2012	2013	*P* Value
Healthy diet education (N = 16,285)	51.22	51.53	49.60	51.17	49.61	53.93	0.04
Physical activity education (N = 16,291)	50.16	49.23	46.84	50.28	48.91	54.90	0.10
Perceived health status: excellent/very good/good (N = 16,316)	78.89	77.13	77.95	80.25	79.45	79.39	0.12
Perceived mental health status: excellent/very good/good (N = 16,315)	89.94	90.01	90.23	90.25	89.56	89.69	0.90
Hospitalization (N = 16,404)	16.16	17.20	16.55	15.56	15.35	16.30	0.44
ER visits (N = 16,404)	18.13	16.67	17.86	16.73	18.65	18.42	0. 20

The actual sample and population size vary because of missing or inapplicable values for different measures

The analyses were weighted to reflect the complex survey design of MEPS

4.7 Analysis

We performed all the data analyses by using Stata/SE 14.0. All the analyses accounted for both the design effect and the sampling weights by using svy command.

(1) Standard descriptive statistics and bivariate relationships

Before any hypothesis testing, initial analyses focused on standard descriptive statistics and bivariate relationships. We described categorical data by using frequencies and percentages. We describe continuous variables in terms of means and standard deviations.

(2) Hypothesis testing

It should be noted that due to the complex sampling design of MEPS, we cannot perform the Chi-square test on weighted data. To get a valid P-value, the Chi-square statistic is converted to an F statistic. The Design-based F test produced by "svy tab" is_ a corrected weighted Pearson Chi-square statistic (StataCorp, 2015). For hypothesis 1.1, we conducted Design-based F tests to compare the likelihood of receiving each of the eight recommended preventive screenings among the patient groups who received PCC, partial PCC and Non-PCC. We performed multivariate logistic regressions to reveal the relationship between the outcome (the receipt of preventive screenings) and the independent variables after control for the covariates. We fit the full model with all possible predictors. Before performing the regressions, we checked if there is a zero in any cell of a 2×2 table for any dichotomous independent and dependent variable in a logistic regression, and prevent the situation that the regressions estimate for the regression coefficient does not exist.

For hypothesis 1.2, we conducted Design-based F tests to compare the likelihood of receiving each of the two types of health education among the patient groups who received PCC, partial PCC and Non-PCC. We then performed multiple logistic regressions to reveal the relationship between the outcome (the receipt of health education) and the associated independent variables after control for the covariates. We fit the full model with all possible predictors.

For hypothesis 2.1, we conducted Design-based F tests to compare the likelihood of patient having good perceived physical and mental health status among the patient groups who received PCC, partial PCC and Non-PCC. We performed multiple logistic regressions to reveal the relationship between the outcome (patient perceived physical health status and mental health status) and the associated independent variables after control for the covariates. We fit the full model with all possible predictors.

For hypothesis 2.2, we conducted Design-based F tests to compare the likelihood of patient having ED visits among the patient groups who received PCC, partial PCC and Non-PCC, and conducted Design-based F test to compare the likelihood of the happening of hospitalization among the three patient groups. We performed multiple logistic models to reveal the relationship between the ED visits and the associated independent variables, and performed multiple logistic regressions to reveal the relationship between the happening of hospitalization and the associated independent variables after control for the covariates. We fit the full model with all possible predictors.

We used standard errors, p-values, odds ratios, and 95% confidence interval to interpret effect size and statistical significance.

References

Aday, L. A., Fleming, G. V., & Andersen, R. (1984). *Access to medical care in the US: Who has it, who doesn't*. Pluribus Press.

Adler, N. E. (1994). Socioeconomic status and health: The challenge of the gradient. *American Psychologist, 49*(1), 15.

Agency for Healthcare Research and Quality. (2009). *Medical expenditure panel survey: Survey background*. Accessed on January 8, 2016. Available at: http://meps.ahrq.gov/mepsweb/about_meps/survey_back.jsp.

Andersen, R. M. (1995). Revisiting the behavioral model and access to medical care: Does it matter? *Journal of Health and Social Behavior, 36*(1), 1–10.

Beal, A., Hernandez, S., & Doty, M. (2009). Latino access to the patient-centered medical home. *Journal of General Internal Medicine, 24*(Suppl 3), 514–520.

Centers for Disease Control and Prevention. (2013b). *The State of Aging and Health in America 2013*. Accessed on January 8, 2016. Available at: http://www.cdc.gov/features/agingandhealth/state_of_aging_and_health_in_america_2013.pdf.

Cohen, J. (1997). Sample design of the medical expenditure panel survey household component. Accessed on January 8, 2016. Available at: http://meps.ahrq.gov/mepsweb/data_files/publications/mr22/mr22.pdf.

Cohen, J. W., Cohen, S. B., & Banthin, J. S. (2009). The medical expenditure panel survey: A national information resource to support healthcare cost research and inform policy and practice. *Medical Care, 47*(7 Suppl 1), S44-50.

Donabedian, A. (1966). Evaluating the quality of medical care. *Milbank Mem Fund Q, 44*(3, Suppl), 166–206.

Donabedian, A. (1988). The quality of care: How can it be assessed? *JAMA, 121*(11), 1145–1150.

Dong, Y., & Peng, J. (2013). Principled missing data methods for researchers. *Springerplus, 2*, 222.

Ellis, P. D. (2010). *The essential guide to effect sizes: An introduction to statistical power, meta-analysis and the interpretation of research results*. https://bitbucket.org/unikum/bibliography/downloads/Ellis.pdf.

Ezzati-Rice, T. M., Rohde, F., & Greenblatt, J. (2008). Sample design of the medical expenditure panel survey household component, 1998–2007. Accessed on January 8, 2016. Available at: http://meps.ahrq.gov/mepsweb/data_files/publications/mr22/mr22.pdf.

Fayers, P. M., & Hand, D. J. (1997). Factor analysis, causal indicators and quality of life. *Quality of Life Research, 6*(2), 139–150.

Heeringa, S. G., West, B. T., & Berglund, P. A. (2010). *Applied survey data analysis*. Chapman & Hall.

Little, R., & Rubin, D. (1989). *Statistical analysis with missing data*. Wiley.

Machlin, S., Yu, W., & Zodet, M. (2005). *Computing standard errors for MEPS estimates*. Accessed on January 8, 2016. Available at: http://www.meps.ahrq.gov/survey_comp/standard_errors.jsp.

Phillips, K. A., Morrison, K. R., Andersen, R., & Aday, L. A. (1998). Understanding the context of healthcare utilization: Assessing environmental and provider-related variables in the behavioral model of utilization. *Health Services Research, 33*(3 Pt 1), 571–596.

Rubin, D. B. (1998). *Multiple imputation of nonresponse in surveys*. Wiley.

Schoen, C., Osborn, R., Doty, M. M., Bishop, M., Peugh, J., & Murukutla, N. (2007). Toward higher-performance health systems: Adults' health care experiences in seven countries, 2007. *Health Affairs (millwood), 26*(6), w717–w734.

StataCorp. (2015). *Stata statistical software: Release 14*. StataCorp LP.

Suhr, D. D. (2005). *Principal component analysis vs. exploratory factor analysis*. Accessed on January 18, 2016. Available at: http://www2.sas.com/proceedings/sugi30/203-30.pdf.

Sullivan, M. D., Leigh, J., & Gaster, B. (2006). Brief report: Training internists in shared decision making about chronic opioid treatment for noncancer pain. *Journal of General Internal Medicine, 21*(4), 360–362.

UCLA Statistical Consulting Group. (2015). *How can I perform a factor analysis with categorical variables*? Accessed on January 8, 2016. Available at: http://www.ats.ucla.edu/stat/stata/faq/efa_categorical.htm

van der Eijk, C., & Rose, J. (2015). Risky business: factor analysis of survey data—Assessing the probability of incorrect dimensionalisation. *PLoS One, 10*(3), e0118900.

van Houwelingen, H. C., Boshuizen, H. C., & Capannesi, M. (2011). Sensitivity analysis of state-transition models: How to deal with a large number of inputs. *Computers in Biology and Medicine, 41*(9), 838–842.

Wagner, E. H., Coleman, K., Reid, R. J., Phillips, K., Abrams, M. K., & Sugarman, J. R. (2012). The changes involved in patient-centered medical home transformation. *Prim Care, 39*(2), 241–259.

Wolff, J. L., Rand-Giovannetti, E., Palmer, S., Wegener, S., Reider, L., Frey, K., Scharfstein, D., & Boult, C. (2009). Caregiving and chronic care: The guided care program for families and friends. *Journals of Gerontology. Series a, Biological Sciences and Medical Sciences, 64*(7), 785–791.

Chapter 5
The Impact of Patient-Centered Care on Preventive Service

5.1 Introduction

This chapter presents the results for the first aims of the study, which assessed the relationship between the receipt of PCC and chronic management, measured by the receipt of preventive screenings and health education for chronic diseases.

The chapter has following sections. It begins by describing the individual's sociodemographic characteristics and system factors of analytic samples as well as the reflected national totals of the population. The chapter then describes the bivariate associations among the study variables. Then we present the results from the logistic regression models, which were used to examine the associations of PCC with chronic condition management while individual sociodemographic and characteristics and system factors were controlled for. The chapter ends with an investigation of the relationships between each PCC attribute and chronic condition management and health outcomes.

5.2 Demographic and Institutional Characteristics

Table 5.1 characterizes the weighted sample for older adults age 65 and above with at least one chronic condition. The final analytic sample size was 16,654. By using the data for persons with a positive person-level weight, the data are used to make estimates for the civilian noninstitutionalized U.S. population for 2009–2013. The weighted population was 181.60 million. The included respondents are adults age 65 and above, who were currently having at least one chronic condition, and having a USC provider. Using the items of PCC in the MEPS, respondents were categorized into three groups: (1) 5963 respondents were grouped into having PCC (those who said yes to all four items in the whole person care domain, has at least one yes in both patient engagement domain and enhanced accessibility domain, and said yes to at least 8 items in total); (2) 6973 respondents were grouped into having partial PCC

H. Liang, *The Impact of Patient-Centered Care*,
https://doi.org/10.1007/978-981-16-3968-5_5

Table 5.1 Sociodemographic and health characteristics: 2009–2013 US Civilian Noninstitutionalized Population Age 65 and above with chronic condition

	Total	Patient-centered care	Partial patient-centered care	Non-patient-centered care	*P*-value
Sample size (unweighted)	16,654	5963	6973	3718	
Weighted population (1000)	181,599.05	64,748.36	76,168.68	40,682.01	
Gender (%)					0.85
Male	43.75	43.95	43.81	43.32	
Female	56.22	56.05	56.19	56.68	
Age (Mean, SE)***	74.29 (0.13)	74.09 (0.18)	74.31 (0.15)	74.56 (0.18)	< 0.001
Race/ethnicity (%)					0.50
Non-Hispanic white only	79.97	79.41	80.61	79.68	
Hispanic	6.90	7.02	6.94	6.65	
Non-Hispanic black only	8.22	8.32	8.16	8.20	
Non-Hispanic Asian only	3.43	3.65	3.12	3.67	
Non-Hispanic other race or multi-race	1.46	1.60	1.17	1.81	
Marital status (%)***					< 0.001
Not married	44.66	41.28	44.65	50.08	
Married	55.34	58.72	55.35	49.92	
Education (%)					0.16
No degree	19.58	18.49	19.75	21.00	
General equivalency diploma/high school diploma	42.68	42.09	42.89	43.22	
Bachelor's degree/some college/associate degree	21.86	22.32	21.90	21.07	
Advance degree	15.88	17.10	15.46	14.71	
Employment status (%)*					0.01
Not employed	80.91	79.16	81.58	82.46	

(continued)

Table 5.1 (continued)

	Total	Patient-centered care	Partial patient-centered care	Non-patient-centered care	*P*-value
Employed	19.09	20.84	18.42	17.54	
Region (%)***					< 0.001
Northeast	19.24	24.10	16.25	17.11	
Midwest	22.67	22.51	23.50	21.37	
South	36.68	33.90	39.22	36.35	
West	21.41	19.49	21.03	25.17	
Household per capita income (Mean, SE)***	31,110.42 (571.89)	32,553.65 (835.17)	30,736.86 (729.93)	29,512.82 (721.31)	< 0.001
Insurance coverage (%)**					0.005
Uninsured	0.71	0.63	0.90	0.46	
Medicare only	36.20	35.88	35.01	38.94	
Medicare and private	52.79	54.12	53.43	49.45	
Medicare and other Public only	9.93	8.88	10.35	10.82	
No medicare and any public/private	0.38	0.50	0.31	0.32	
Need help with ADLs (%)					0.13
No	93.09	93.15	93.55	92.13	
Yes	6.91	6.85	6.45	7.87	
Need help with IADLs (%)*					0.04
No	88.45	88.99	88.87	86.81	
Yes	11.55	11.01	11.13	13.19	
Chronic conditions					
Number of chronic conditions (Mean, SE)***	3.91 (0.02)	3.92 (0.04)	3.92 (0.03)	3.91 (0.04)	< 0.001
% Multiple conditions (≥2 conditions) (%)	90.92	90.43	91.48	90.66	0.25

(continued)

Table 5.1 (continued)

	Total	Patient-centered care	Partial patient-centered care	Non-patient-centered care	*P*-value
% ≥ 5 Conditions (%)	34.60	34.67	34.43	34.82	0.95
Provider's type (%)***					< 0.001
Facility	36.67	40.84	34.64	33.82	
Person	32.61	32.30	33.49	31.47	
Person in facility provider	30.72	26.86	31.88	34.71	
Provider's location (%)***					< 0.001
Office	82.69	80.73	84.42	82.57	
Hospital, not ER	17.31	19.27	15.58	17.43	

*$p < 0.05$ **$p < 0.01$, ***$p < 0.001$ based on t test continuous measures and design-based F test for categorical measures
The standard errors of all survey estimates and associated test statistics have been adjusted for the impact of clustering due to the complex multistage survey design and unequal weighting

(those who said yes to all four items in the whole person care domain, has at least one yes in both patient engagement domain and enhanced accessibility domain); (3) 3718 respondents were grouped into Non-PCC (those who said no to any of four items in the whole person care domain, or has no in patient engagement domain and/or enhanced accessibility domain). Table 5.1 shows the samples size, number of weighted population for the each group and the weighted percentage of each characteristic.

Overall, 56% of the sample was female. The mean age of included respondents was 74 ± 0.13 years. In terms of predisposing factors, there were no significant differences among the three groups in race/ethnicity and education level distributions. The majority of the respondents were non-Hispanic Whites (80%). About 42% of respondents' highest degrees were high school. Compared with PCC and partial PCC samples, the non-PCC sample included more unmarried (50%) and unemployed people (82%). For the whole sample, a higher proportion of respondents lived in the South (37%) and a smaller percentage in the Northeast (19%). The proportion of West respondents in non-PCC group was higher than PCC and partial PCC group.

In terms of enabling factors, the household per capita income were higher in PCC and partial PCC respondents than the non-PCC respondents. Respondents from PCC and partial PCC groups had higher rate of Medicare and Private insurance coverage, whereas non-PCC respondents were more likely to be only covered through Medicare.

With respect to needs factors, there were no significant differences among the three groups in needs of IADL and the number of chronic conditions. Respondents from all the three groups were having around four chronic conditions. More than 90% of respondents had multiple conditions, and more than 34% of respondents had five or over five chronic conditions. There were differences in system factors among three groups. In terms of the variable of provider's type, providers in PCC group were more likely to be facilities (41%), while providers in partial and non-PCC groups were more likely to be persons in facilities (35 and 34% respectively). As for the variable of provider's location, more proportion of partial PCC and non-PCC's provider were located in office (84 and 83% respectively), while this proportion of PCC group were 81%.

All these demographic and institutional characteristics were controlled in the multivariate logistic regressions.

5.3 Bivariate Results

In this section, the bivariate results for aim 1 and 2 of this study are presented respectively, which assessed the associations between the receipt of PCC and ten preventive care measures as well as four health outcome measures, and test the hypotheses that if the receipt of PCC will increase the likelyhood of receiving preventive services as well as health outcome measures for chronic conditions.

Table 5.2 presents the bivariate associations between PCC status and the proportions of receiving preventive care. Overall, the results of each comparison were significant at $P < 0.05$. There were significant differences in receiving eight preventive screenings and two types of health education across the three groups. Among the three groups of respondents, the PCC respondents had the highest proportions in eight out of ten measures, followed by the partial PCC group. The non-PCC group reported the lowest proportions of receiving each of the ten preventive care services.

Among the six measures reported by both male and female respondents, more than 97% of patients received blood pressure check, and more than 91% of patients received cholesterol check and routine checkup within the past 12 month. In contrast, the rate of receiving blood stool test within the past year ranked last with a proportion of 18.8%. As for the three preventive care measures for female, more than 95% of the female respondents reported that they had ever received Pap smear test, around 60% of the female respondents reported that they had received breast exam within the past 12 month, and around 74% of the female respondents reported that they had received mammogram test within the past 24 months. As for the preventive care measures for male, 69% of the male respondents reported that they had ever received PSA tests before. Finally, with regard to the both health education interventions (i.e. healthy diet and physical activity), the proportions for both measures were beyond 50%. The results from our study were relatively higher than the nationwide data reported by the related national institutes, because the included respondents in our study were those older chronic disease patients who had usual source of care. Studies showed people having usual source of care were more likely to receive preventive services than the general population (Shi, 2012; Tsai et al., 2010). Here are the related data

Table 5.2 Preventive care and health education rates: comparisons between patient-centered care patients and non patient-centered care patients

	Total	Patient-centered care	Partial patient-centered care	Non-patient-centered care	*P* Value
		% (95% CI)			
Sample size (Unweighted)	16,654	5963	6973	3718	
Weighted population (1000)	181,599.05	64,748.36	76,168.68	40,682.01	
Blood pressure check within the previous 12 months (N = 16,283)	97.57 (97.23, 97.86)	97.59 (96.05, 98.03)	97.89 (97.40, 98.28)	96.94 (96.15,97.57)	0.04
Cholesterol check within the previous 12 months (N = 16,283)	91.66 (90.91, 92.35)	93.44 (92.34, 94.39)	92.33 (91.34, 93.22)	87.58 (85.84, 89.14)	< 0.001
Routine checkup within the previous 12 months (N = 16,283)	91.11 (90.22, 91.93)	93.09 (92.03, 94.03)	91.28 (90.06, 92.36)	87.64 (85.89, 89.20)	< 0.001
Blood stool test within the previous 12 months (N = 16,259)	18.81 (17.47, 20.24)	21.23 (19.51, 23.25)	19.88 (18.04, 21.85)	12.83 (11.34, 14.48)	< 0.001
Breast exam within the previous 12 months (only for women) (N = 9347)	59.61 (58.04, 61.17)	62.94 (60.68, 65.15)	60.82 (58.74, 62.85)	52.16 (49.24, 55.06)	< 0.001
Mammogram within the previous 24 months (only for women) (N = 9348)	73.55 (72.15, 74.91)	75.90 (73.94, 77.77)	74.83 (72.79, 76.77)	67.48 (64.76, 70.10)	< 0.001

(continued)

Table 5.2 (continued)

	Total	Patient-centered care	Partial patient-centered care	Non-patient-centered care	*P* Value
		% (95% CI)			
Pap smear test (only for women) (N = 9344)	95.99 (95.35, 96.54)	97.18 (96.37, 97.82)	97.64 (96.93, 98.19)	91.04 (89.12, 92.65)	< 0.001
PSA test (only for men) (N = 6900)	68.65 (66.95, 70.30)	71.25 (68.73, 73.65)	71.20 (69.14, 73.17)	59.61 (56.44, 62.70)	< 0.001
Healthy diet education (N = 16,285)	51.22 (49.65, 52.78)	54.82 (52.70, 56.92)	50.03 (47.97, 52.10)	47.71 (45.46, 49.97)	< 0.001
Physical activity education (N = 16,291)	50.16 (48.71, 51.60)	53.29 (51.25, 55.32)	48.63 (46.62, 50.65)	48.05 (45.89, 50.20)	< 0.001

The estimates and associated test statistics have been adjusted for the impact of clustering due to the complex multistage survey design and unequal weighting

The actual sample and population size vary because of missing or inapplicable values for different measures

of the whole US population: blood stool test within the past 12 months: 65.1% (50–75 years old, CDC, 2012); mammography within the past 24 months: 61% (65 and older, CDC, 2012); ever had a Pap smear test: 69.4% (18 and older, CDC, 2013); and ever had a PSA test:51.2% (60–74 years old, CDC, 2010).

As for the comparison among the three groups, the PCC and the partial PCC patients were significantly more likely to receive each of the eight preventive screenings as well as the two types of health education. The PCC respondents reported remarkable higher proportion of receiving blood stool test, breast exam and PSA test than non-PCC respondents. The magnitude of differences between the PCC group and the non-PCC group in these three measures reached 10%. The difference between the PCC group and the non-PCC group in blood pressure check within the previous 12 months was small (97.6% vs. 96.9%). In terms of the other 6 measures, the proportions of PCC group were 5–8% higher than the proportions of the non-PCC group. Notably, the differences of proportions in six preventive screening measures between PCC group and the partial PCC group were small, ranged from 0.05 to 2.12%. The differences between the PCC group and the partial PCC group in two health education measures (healthy diet education and physical activity education) were 4.79 and 4.66%.

5.4 Multivariate Results

5.4.1 Multivariate Analysis: PCC Status Associated with Preventive Screening and Health Education

Table 5.3 displays the multiple logistic regression results associating the receipt of PCC with preventive care measures after control for individual predisposing, enabling, and need covariates as well as system covariates. The results relate the status of PCC (PCC vs. non-PCC and partial PCC vs. non-PCC) to the odds of receiving preventive care. Both the odds ratios and their 95% confidence intervals are presented. Similar to the findings from the bivariate analyses, even after control for individual and institutional characteristics, the PCC group was found to be more likely than the non-PCC group to receive seven types of preventive screenings and two types of health education, and the partial PCC group was found to be more likely than the non-PCC group to receive eight types of preventive screenings.

As for the eight preventive screening measures, the PCC status was associated with higher odds in getting seven types of preventive screenings, while partial PCC was associated with higher odds in getting all the eight preventive screenings. Specifically, the PCC group was 1.99 (95% CI: 1.58–2.51, $P < 0.001$) times more likely than the non-PCC group to get cholesterol checks within the previous 12 months, was 1.84 (95% CI: 1.51–2.24, $P < 0.001$) times more likely than the non-PCC group to get routine checkups within the previous 12 months, was 1.87 (95% CI: 1.58–2.21, $P < 0.001$) times more likely than the non-PCC group to get blood stool test within the previous 12 months, was 1.45 (95% CI: 1.25–1.68, $P < 0.001$) times more likely than the non-PCC group to get breast exam within the previous 12 months, was 1.38 (95% CI: 1.18–1.63, $P < 0.001$) times more likely than the non-PCC group to get mammogram within the previous 24 months, was 3.19 (95% CI: 2.29–4.43, $P < 0.001$) times more likely than the non-PCC group to receive Pap smear test, and was 1.62 (95% CI: 1.38–2.89, $P < 0.001$) times more likely than non-PCC group to get PSA test.

Similarly, the partial PCC group also performed better than the non-PCC group, which was associated with higher odds in getting all the eight preventive screenings than the non-PCC group. Specifically, the partial PCC group was 1.44 (95% CI: 1.05–1.99, $P < 0.05$) times more likely than the non-PCC group to get blood pressure checks within the previous 12 months, was 1.67 (95% CI: 1.37–2.03, $P < 0.001$) times more likely than the non-PCC group to get cholesterol checks within the previous 12 months, was 1.46 (95% CI: 1.23–1.73, $P < 0.001$) times more likely than the non-PCC group to get routine checkups within the previous 12 months, was 1.72 (95% CI: 1.49–1.98, $P < 0.001$) times more likely than the non-PCC group to get blood stool test within the previous 12 months, was 1.36 (95% CI: 1.19–1.55, $P < 0.001$) times more likely than the non-PCC group to get breast exam within the previous 12 months, was 1.33 (95% CI: 1.15–1.54, $P < 0.001$) times more likely than the non-PCC group to get mammogram within the previous 24 months, was 3.90 (95% CI: 2.81–5.41, $P < 0.001$) times more likely than the non-PCC group to receive Pap

Table 5.3 Multivariate analysis of correlates of preventive care and health education rates

	Preventive care				
	Blood pressure check within the previous 12 months (N = 16,283)	Cholesterol check within the previous 12 months (N = 16,283)	Routine checkup within the previous 12 months (N = 16,283)	Blood stool test within the previous 12 months (N = 16,259)	Breast exam within the previous 12 months (for women only) (N = 9347)
			OR (95% CI)		
Patient-centered care					
Non-PCC	Ref.	Ref.	Ref.	Ref.	Ref.
Partial-PCC	1.44 (1.05, 1.99)*	1.67 (1.37, 2.03)***	1.46 (1.23, 1.73)***	1.72 (1.49, 1.98)***	1.36 (1.19, 1.55)***
PCC	1.28 (0.92, 1.77)	1.99 (1.58, 2.51)***	1.84 (1.51, 2.24)***	1.87 (1.58, 2.21)***	1.45 (1.25, 1.68)***
Gender					
Male	Ref.	Ref.	Ref.	Ref.	–
Female	1.08 (0.83, 1.40)	0.86 (0.74, 0.99)*	0.95 (0.83, 1.10)	0.84 (0.76, 0.92)***	–
Age	1.02 (1.00, 1.04)	1.00 (0.99, 1.02)	1.02 (1.01, 1.03)**	1.00 (0.99, 1.01)	0.96 (0.95, 0.97)***
Race/ethnicity					
Non-Hispanic white only	Ref.	Ref.	Ref.	Ref.	Ref.
Hispanic	1.03 (0.68, 1.55)	1.63 (1.26, 2.11)***	1.29 (0.92, 1.80)	1.55 (1.27, 1.88)***	1.21 (1.01, 1.46)*
Non-Hispanic black only	1.09 (0.75, 1.58)	1.39 (1.09, 1.77)**	1.78 (1.40, 2.25)***	1.38 (1.19, 1.61)***	1.51 (1.27, 1.80)***
Non-Hispanic Asian only	0.99 (0.61, 1.60)	1.65 (1.28, 2.14)***	1.59 (1.14, 2.22)**	1.37 (1.10, 1.72)**	0.86 (0.69, 1.07)
Non-Hispanic other race or multi-race	1.07 (0.46, 2.50)	1.12 (0.66, 1.88)	1.66 (0.98, 2.82)	0.94 (0.66, 1.34)	1.25 (0.86, 1.80)
Marital status					
Not married	Ref.	Ref.	Ref.	Ref.	Ref.
Married	1.17 (0.89, 1.53)	1.27 (1.07, 1.51)**	1.16 (0.97, 1.39)	1.13 (0.98, 1.29)	1.23 (1.09, 1.38)**
Education					
No degree	Ref.	Ref.	Ref.	Ref.	Ref.

(continued)

Table 5.3 (continued)

	Preventive care				
	Blood pressure check within the previous 12 months (N = 16,283)	Cholesterol check within the previous 12 months (N = 16,283)	Routine checkup within the previous 12 months (N = 16,283)	Blood stool test within the previous 12 months (N = 16,259)	Breast exam within the previous 12 months (for women only) (N = 9347)
			OR (95% CI)		
General equivalency diploma/high school diploma	1.20 (0.85, 1.71)	1.09 (0.87, 1.36)	1.25 (1.03, 1.52)*	1.18 (1.02, 1.36)*	1.27 (1.08, 1.48)**
Bachelor's degree/some college/associate degree	1.70 (1.13, 2.57)*	1.42 (1.09, 1.85)**	1.56 (1.19, 2.04)**	1.29 (1.08, 1.52)**	1.45 (1.22, 1.72)***
Advance degree	1.97 (1.20, 3.21)**	1.35 (1.00, 1.82)*	1.37 (1.02, 1.85)*	1.28 (1.05, 1.56)*	1.36 (1.10, 1.68)**
Employment status					
Not employed	Ref.	Ref.	Ref.	Ref.	Ref.
Employed	0.65 (0.46, 0.93)*	0.72 (0.58, 0.89)**	0.75 (0.60, 0.92)**	0.91 (0.76, 1.08)	0.94 (0.79, 1.11)
Region					
Northeast	Ref.	Ref.	Ref.	Ref.	Ref.
Midwest	0.66 (0.42, 1.03)	0.77 (0.57, 1.05)	0.50 (0.38, 0.67)***	0.93 (0.74, 1.17)	0.95 (0.76, 1.17)
South	0.80 (0.52, 1.24)	1.03 (0.77, 1.39)	0.61 (0.45, 0.82)**	1.22 (0.96, 1.56)	0.83 (0.69, 0.99)*
West	0.66 (0.43, 1.04)	0.65 (0.47, 0.88)**	0.47 (0.36, 0.62)***	1.50 (1.22, 1.85)***	0.85 (0.69, 1.04)
Household per capita income					
0–9999	Ref.	Ref.	Ref.	Ref.	Ref.
10,000–24,999	1.33 (0.97, 1.82)	1.18 (0.98, 1.43)	1.21 (1.01, 1.45)*	1.08 (0.94, 1.23)	1.01 (0.87, 1.17)
25,000–49,999	1.44 (0.96, 2.16)	1.28 (1.01, 1.63)*	1.42 (1.11, 1.82)**	1.02 (0.86, 1.21)	1.27 (1.06, 1.51)**
50,000 or more	1.86 (1.17, 2.95)**	1.48 (1.08, 2.02)*	1.50 (1.13, 2.00)**	1.22 (0.97, 1.55)	1.49 (1.20, 1.84)***
Insurance coverage					

(continued)

Table 5.3 (continued)

	Preventive care				
	Blood pressure check within the previous 12 months (N = 16,283)	Cholesterol check within the previous 12 months (N = 16,283)	Routine checkup within the previous 12 months (N = 16,283)	Blood stool test within the previous 12 months (N = 16,259)	Breast exam within the previous 12 months (for women only) (N = 9347)
			OR (95% CI)		
Uninsured	Ref.	Ref.	Ref.	Ref.	Ref.
Medicare only	1.68 (0.90, 3.13)	1.32 (0.73, 2.38)	1.79 (1.04, 3.05)*	1.38 (0.80, 2.40)	0.73 (0.42, 1.27)
Medicare and private	2.33 (1.19, 4.56)*	1.55 (0.85, 2.82)	2.00 (1.19, 3.38)**	1.21 (0.70, 2.09)	0.94 (0.54, 1.64)
Medicare and other public only	2.41 (1.32, 4.38)**	1.77 (0.96, 3.28)	1.80 (1.04, 3.11)*	1.38 (0.79, 2.42)	0.78 (0.44, 1.38)
No medicare and any public/private	0.96 (0.25, 3.69)	0.60 (0.17, 2.12)	1.17 (0.43, 3.18)	0.59 (0.18, 1.93)	1.26 (0.48, 3.33)
Need help with ADLs					
No	Ref.	Ref.	Ref.	Ref.	Ref.
Yes	1.61 (0.64, 4.02)	0.92 (0.65, 1.32)	0.85 (0.60, 1.21)	1.17 (0.90, 1.52)	0.93 (0.74, 1.17)
Need help with IADLs					
No	Ref.	Ref.	Ref.	Ref.	Ref.
Yes	1.04 (0.58, 1.86)	0.77 (0.58, 1.03)	0.80 (0.60, 1.07)	1.08 (0.87, 1.34)	0.70 (0.57, 0.85)***
Number of chronic conditions	1.61 (1.46, 1.79)***	1.47 (1.40, 1.54)***	1.29 (1.24, 1.35)***	1.06 (1.03, 1.08)***	1.02 (0.99, 1.06)
Provider's type					
Facility	Ref.	Ref.	Ref.	Ref.	Ref.
Person	1.01 (0.73, 1.39)	1.24 (1.01, 1.53)*	1.25 (1.03, 1.51)*	0.98 (0.82, 1.16)	1.20 (1.02, 1.40)*
Person in facility Provider	1.48 (1.08, 2.01)*	1.21 (0.99, 1.47)	1.16 (0.98, 1.37)	0.88 (0.75, 1.03)	1.09 (0.95, 1.26)
Provider's location					
Office	Ref.	Ref.	Ref.	Ref.	Ref.
Hospital, not ER	0.69 (0.49, 0.96)*	1.03 (0.82, 1.28)	0.88 (0.74, 1.06)	1.23 (1.08, 1.41)**	1.02 (0.86, 1.21)

(continued)

Table 5.3 (continued)

	Preventive care				
	Blood pressure check within the previous 12 months (N = 16,283)	Cholesterol check within the previous 12 months (N = 16,283)	Routine checkup within the previous 12 months (N = 16,283)	Blood stool test within the previous 12 months (N = 16,259)	Breast exam within the previous 12 months (for women only) (N = 9347)
			OR (95% CI)		
Patient-centered care					
Non-PCC	Ref.	Ref.	Ref.	Ref.	Ref.
Partial-PCC	1.33 (1.15, 1.54)***	3.90 (2.81, 5.41)***	1.63 (1.40, 1.90)***	1.08 (0.95, 1.21)	1.00 (0.89, 1.14)
PCC	1.38 (1.18, 1.63)***	3.19 (2.29, 4.43)***	1.62 (1.38, 1.89)***	1.30 (1.15, 1.47)***	1.21 (1.07, 1.37)**
Gender					
Male	–	–	–	Ref.	Ref.
Female	–	–	–	0.94 (0.86, 1.03)	1.02 (0.94, 1.11)
Age	0.94 (0.93, 0.95)***	0.94 (0.92, 0.97)***	0.99 (0.97, 0.99)*	0.95 (0.94, 0.96)***	0.95 (0.94, 0.95)***
Race/ethnicity					
Non-Hispanic white only	Ref.	Ref.	Ref.	Ref.	Ref.
Hispanic	1.42 (1.13, 1.78)**	0.86 (0.56, 1.33)	0.89 (0.71, 1.10)	2.15 (1.86, 2.49)***	2.11 (1.82, 2.44)***
Non-Hispanic black only	1.38 (1.13, 1.68)**	0.91 (0.62, 1.33)	1.12 (0.90, 1.38)	1.34 (1.17, 1.54)***	1.41 (1.23, 1.61)***
Non-Hispanic Asian only	0.74 (0.58, 0.95)*	0.25 (0.16, 0.41)***	0.58 (0.43, 0.80)**	1.61 (1.25, 2.08)***	1.63 (1.32, 2.02)***
Non-Hispanic other race or multi-race	0.92 (0.49, 1.73)	1.69 (0.57, 5.08)	0.74 (0.47, 1.17)	1.11 (0.77, 1.60)	1.42 (0.98, 2.05)
Marital status					
Not married					
Married	1.46 (1.26, 1.69)***	1.00 (0.73, 1.37)	1.29 (1.09, 1.52)**	1.14 (1.03, 1.26)*	1.10 (1.00, 1.21)
Education					
No degree	Ref.	Ref.	Ref.	Ref.	Ref.

(continued)

Table 5.3 (continued)

	Preventive care				
	Blood pressure check within the previous 12 months (N = 16,283)	Cholesterol check within the previous 12 months (N = 16,283)	Routine checkup within the previous 12 months (N = 16,283)	Blood stool test within the previous 12 months (N = 16,259)	Breast exam within the previous 12 months (for women only) (N = 9347)
			OR (95% CI)		
General equivalency diploma/high school diploma	1.39 (1.16, 1.66)***	1.13 (0.81, 1.56)	1.51 (1.26, 1.80)***	0.97 (0.87, 1.08)	1.10 (0.97, 1.24)
Bachelor's degree/some college/associate degree	1.47 (1.18, 1.83)**	1.89 (1.11, 3.20)*	1.47 (1.15, 1.88)**	0.94 (0.82, 1.08)	1.23 (1.07, 1.42)**
Advance degree	1.80 (1.32, 2.45)***	1.18 (0.69, 2.02)	1.43 (1.11, 1.84)**	0.93 (0.80, 1.07)	1.08 (0.92, 1.28)
Employment status					
Not Employed	Ref.	Ref.	Ref.	Ref.	Ref.
Employed	1.16 (0.89, 1.49)	0.76 (0.47, 1.23)	0.97 (0.81, 1.16)	0.98 (0.85, 1.14)	0.91 (0.79, 1.04)
Region					
Northeast	Ref.	Ref.	Ref.	Ref.	Ref.
Midwest	0.98 (0.76, 1.25)	0.92 (0.53, 1.60)	0.90 (0.71, 1.14)	0.89 (0.75, 1.06)	0.90 (0.75, 1.08)
South	1.00 (0.79, 1.26)	1.10 (0.73, 1.67)	0.98 (0.77, 1.24)	0.98 (0.85, 1.13)	0.96 (0.82, 1.13)
West	0.97 (0.76, 1.24)	1.27 (0.81, 1.99)	0.79 (0.60, 1.05)	0.88 (0.72, 1.08)	0.96 (0.81, 1.14)
Household per capita income					
0–9999	Ref.	Ref.	Ref.	Ref.	Ref.
10,000–24,999	1.07 (0.91, 1.26)	1.17 (0.87, 1.57)	0.99 (0.82, 1.19)	1.03 (0.90, 1.18)	1.04 (0.90, 1.19)
25,000–49,999	1.33 (1.10, 1.61)**	1.43 (0.95, 2.16)	1.27 (1.02, 1.60)*	1.06 (0.92, 1.22)	1.06 (0.92, 1.22)
50,000 or more	1.62 (1.24, 2.12)**	1.45 (0.87, 2.39)	1.34 (1.05, 1.72)*	1.17 (0.98, 1.41)	1.11 (0.90, 1.35)
Insurance coverage					

(continued)

Table 5.3 (continued)

	Preventive care				
	Blood pressure check within the previous 12 months (N = 16,283)	Cholesterol check within the previous 12 months (N = 16,283)	Routine checkup within the previous 12 months (N = 16,283)	Blood stool test within the previous 12 months (N = 16,259)	Breast exam within the previous 12 months (for women only) (N = 9347)
			OR (95% CI)		
Uninsured	Ref.	Ref.	Ref.	Ref.	Ref.
Medicare only	2.45 (1.26, 4.78)**	1.68 (0.58, 4.87)	1.50 (0.87, 2.59)	1.25 (0.88, 1.77)	1.40 (0.99, 1.97)
Medicare and private	3.23 (1.65, 6.32)**	2.80 (0.97, 8.12)	1.71 (1.00, 2.95)	1.27 (0.90, 1.80)	1.47 (1.04, 2.10)*
Medicare and other public only	2.39 (1.22, 4.69)*	1.42 (0.49, 4.11)	1.53 (0.87, 2.69)	1.23 (0.84, 1.80)	1.39 (0.96, 2.03)
No medicare and any public/private	1.30 (0.39, 4.32)	1.66 (0.20, 13.86)	0.77 (0.32, 1.88)	1.03 (0.43, 2.49)	1.20 (0.55, 2.62)
Need help with ADLs					
No	Ref.	Ref.	Ref.	Ref.	Ref.
Yes	0.63 (0.50, 0.80)***	0.82 (0.50, 1.35)	1.02 (0.75, 1.39)	0.92 (0.74, 1.14)	0.74 (0.58, 0.94)*
Need help with IADLs					
No	Ref.	Ref.	Ref.	Ref.	Ref.
Yes	0.68 (0.56, 0.83)***	0.64 (0.40, 1.02)	0.73 (0.56, 0.95)**	0.86 (0.73, 1.01)	0.86 (0.73, 1.02)
Number of Chronic Conditions	1.05 (1.01, 1.09)**	1.10 (1.02, 1.19)*	1.04 (1.00, 1.08)	1.32 (1.29, 1.36)***	1.26 (1.23, 1.30)***
Provider's type					
Facility	Ref.	Ref.	Ref.	Ref.	Ref.
Person	1.19 (1.00, 1.41)*	0.93 (0.65, 1.35)	1.36 (1.13, 1.63)**	1.08 (0.95, 1.23)	1.07 (0.95, 1.22)
Person in facility Provider	1.09 (0.95, 1.25)	0.89 (0.61, 1.28)	1.10 (0.92, 1.30)	1.03 (0.91, 1.16)	1.18 (1.05, 1.33)**
Provider's location					
Office	Ref.	Ref.	Ref.	Ref.	Ref.
hospital, not ER	0.99 (0.80, 1.23)	0.94 (0.65, 1.38)	1.02 (0.86, 1.22)	1.02 (0.90, 1.16)	1.05 (0.91, 1.21)

$*p < 0.05$, $**p < 0.01$, $***p < 0.001$

The analyses were weighted to reflect the complex survey design of MEPS

smear test, and was 1.63 (95% CI: 1.40–1.90, $P < 0.001$) times more likely than the non-PCC group to get PSA test.

In terms of health education measures, PCC status was significantly associated with higher odds in getting the two types of health educations. Specifically, PCC group was 1.30 (95% CI: 1.15–1.47, $P < 0.001$) times more likely than the non-PCC group to receive healthy diet education, and was 1.21 (95% CI: 1.07–1.37, $P < 0.01$) times more likely than the non-PCC group to get routine checkups within the previous 12 months.

Finally, with regard to the comparisons for magnitude of OR, the results showed that there were no significant differences between PCC and partial PCC in the terms of ORs compare to non-PCC. Among the ten measures, the highest magnitude of OR was found for the measure of Pap smear test. Both PCC and partial PCC group had more than three times the odds of receiving Pap smear test than the non-PCC group.

The significant associations between other predictor variables of interest and preventive care measures were also observed. As for the predisposing factors, the results showed that women were less likely than men to receive cholesterol checks (OR: 0.86, 95% CI: 0.74–0.99) and blood stool test (OR: 0.84, 95% CI: 0.76–0.92) within the previous 12 months. Moreover, a year older age was associated with a 2% higher odds of receiving routine checkups (OR: 1.02, 95% CI: 1.01–1.03). As for the race/ethnicity, the results showed the receipt of preventive care services varied according to the PCC status. Other variables, such as the married status and higher education level, were also found to be more likely to receive specific types of preventive care. In terms of the enabling factors, household per capital income level of USD 50,000 was significantly associated with higher odds in getting six types of preventive screening services, and the level of USD 25,000–49,000 was significantly associated with higher odds in getting five types of preventive screenings. Notably, the results showed that the receipt of blood stool tests and Pap smear tests were not associated with the household per capita income level. The results also showed that respondents who were covered by Medicare plus private insurance were associated with higher odds of receiving blood pressure tests, routine checkups and mammograms. Regarding the needs covariates, the need help with ADLs was associated with lower odds of receiving mammography and exercise education, while the need help with IADL was associated with lower odds of receiving breast exam, mammography and PSA tests. An elevated number of chronic conditions was significantly associated with higher odds of receiving six types of preventive screenings and two types of health education. Finally, with regard to the system factors, the results showed that patients who visited person type providers (e.g. family physicians, primary care doctor in doctor's office rather than hospitals or ER) were more associated with higher odds of providing five types of preventive screening.

5.4.2 PCC Attributes Associated with Receiving Preventive Screening and Health Education

Before we performing the multiple logistic regression to explore the association between the PCC attributes with preventive screening and health education measures, we used the user-written Stata command Collin to exam the tolerance and the Variance Inflation Factor (VIF) of predictor variables. The severity of collinearity in an ordinary least squares (OLS) regression analysis can be measured by the VIF, which produces an index that quantifies how much the variance of an estimated regression coefficient is increased because of collinearity (Greene, 2000). Results from the multicollinearity test showed results in VIF scores ranging from 1.01 to 2.59. Since the VIF for all of our independent variables are less than 10, we concluded that there were no unacceptable biases caused by the correlations among the independent variables.

Table 5.4 displays the multiple logistic regression results associating PCC attributes with preventive screening and health education measures after control for individual predisposing, enabling, and need covariates as well as system covariates. The results relate the attributes of PCC (whole person care vs. non- whole person care, patient engagement vs. non-patient engagement and enhanced access vs. non-enhanced access) to the odds of receiving preventive care. Both the odds ratios and their 95% confidence intervals are presented.

As for preventive screening measures, the whole person care attribute of PCC was associated with higher odds in getting seven out of eight types of preventive screenings; the patient engagement attribute was associated with higher odds in getting six out of eight preventive screenings; and the enhanced access attributes was associated with higher odds in getting two out of eight preventive screenings. Specifically, the patient who were having whole person care was 1.94 (95% CI: 1.26–2.98, $P < 0.01$) times more likely to get the blood pressure check within the previous 12 months than the patient who were not having whole person care, was 2.11 (95% CI: 1.48–3.00, $P < 0.001$) times more likely to get cholesterol checks within the previous 12 months, was 2.04 (95% CI: 1.49- 2.79, $P < 0.001$) times more likely to get routine checkups within the previous 12 months, was 1.47 (95% CI: 1.08–2.00, $P < 0.05$) times more likely to get the blood stool test within the previous 12 months, was 1.35 (95% CI: 1.02–1.79, $P < 0.05$) times more to get the breast exam within the previous 12 months, was 2.45 (95% CI: 1.47–4.08, $P < 0.01$) times more likely to receive the Pap smear test, and was 1.75 (95% CI: 1.29–2.38, $P < 0.001$) times more likely to get the PSA test.

Similarly, patient engagement attribute was also associated with higher odds in getting six types of preventive screenings. Specifically, the patient who got patient engagement was 1.29 (95% CI: 1.12–1.49, $P < 0.01$) times more likely to cholesterol checks within the previous 12 months than the patient who did not get patient engagement, was 1.30 (95% CI: 1.13- 1.49, $P < 0.01$) times more likely to get routine checkups within the previous 12 months, was 1.15 (95% CI: 1.04–1.27, $P < 0.01$) times more likely to get the breast exam within the previous 12 months, was 1.14

Table 5.4 Multivariate analysis of correlates of PCC attributes with preventive care and health education rates

	Preventive care				
	Blood pressure check within the previous 12 months (N = 14,643)	Cholesterol check within the previous 12 months (N = 14,341)	Routine checkup within the previous 12 months (N = 14,528)	Blood stool test within the previous 12 months (N = 13,820)	Breast exam within the previous 12 months (for women only) (N = 8025)
			OR (95% CI)		
PCC attributes					
Whole person care					
No	Ref.	Ref.	Ref.	Ref.	Ref.
Yes	1.94 (1.26, 2.98)**	2.11 (1.48, 3.00)***	2.04 (1.49, 2.79)***	1.47 (1.08, 2.00)*	1.35 (1.02, 1.79)*
Patient Engagement and shared decision making					
No	Ref.	Ref.	Ref.	Ref.	Ref.
Yes	1.07 (0.83, 1.36)	1.29 (1.12, 1.49)**	1.30 (1.13, 1.49)***	1.07 (0.95, 1.21)	1.15 (1.04, 1.27)**
Accessible care					
No	Ref.	Ref.	Ref.	Ref.	Ref.
Yes	0.83 (0.61, 1.14)	1.14 (0.90, 1.44)	1.07 (0.86, 1.32)	1.36 (1.17, 1.58)***	1.00 (0.85, 1.18)
Gender					
Male	Ref.	Ref.	Ref.	Ref.	–
Female	1.08 (0.83, 1.40)	0.86 (0.75, 1.00)*	0.96 (0.84, 1.10)	0.85 (0.77, 0.93)**	–
Age	1.02 (1.00, 1.04)	1.00 (0.99, 1.02)	1.02 (1.01, 1.03)**	1.00 (0.99, 1.01)	0.96 (0.95, 0.97)***
Race/ethnicity					
Non-Hispanic white only	Ref.	Ref.	Ref.	Ref.	Ref.
Hispanic	1.03 (0.68, 1.56)	1.67 (1.29, 2.16)***	1.31 (0.94, 1.84)	1.57 (1.29, 1.91)***	1.22 (1.02, 1.47)*
Non-Hispanic black only	1.09 (0.74, 1.58)	1.39 (1.09, 1.78)**	1.79 (1.41, 2.27)***	1.37 (1.18, 1.60)***	1.51 (1.28, 1.80)***
Non-Hispanic Asian only	0.99 (0.61, 1.60)	1.67 (1.29, 2.16)***	1.63 (1.17, 2.29)**	1.35 (1.09, 1.68)**	0.87 (0.70, 1.09)
Non-Hispanic other race or multi-race	1.03 (0.44, 2.46)	1.07 (0.63, 1.81)	1.61 (0.94, 2.76)	0.91 (0.64, 1.31)	1.23 (0.85, 1.77)

(continued)

Table 5.4 (continued)

	Preventive care				
	Blood pressure check within the previous 12 months (N = 14,643)	Cholesterol check within the previous 12 months (N = 14,341)	Routine checkup within the previous 12 months (N = 14,528)	Blood stool test within the previous 12 months (N = 13,820)	Breast exam within the previous 12 months (for women only) (N = 8025)
			OR (95% CI)		
Marital status					
Not married	Ref.	Ref.	Ref.	Ref.	Ref.
Married	1.16 (0.89, 1.52)	1.27 (1.07, 1.51)**	1.16 (0.96, 1.39)	1.14 (0.99, 1.30)	1.22 (1.09, 1.38)**
Education					
No degree	Ref.	Ref.	Ref.	Ref.	Ref.
General equivalency diploma/high school diploma	1.21 (0.85, 1.72)	1.10 0.88, 1.37)	1.26 (1.04, 1.53)*	1.19 (1.03, 1.37)*	1.27 (1.08, 1.48)**
Bachelor's degree/some college/associate degree	1.71 (1.13, 2.58)*	1.44 (1.11, 1.87)**	1.57 (1.21, 2.05)**	1.30 (1.10, 1.54)**	1.45 (1.22, 1.73)***
Advance degree	1.98 (1.21, 3.23)**	1.36 (1.00, 1.83)*	1.37 (1.02, 1.85)*	1.29 (1.06, 1.57)*	1.35 (1.10, 1.68)**
Employment status					
Not Employed	Ref.	Ref.	Ref.	Ref.	Ref.
Employed	0.65 (0.46, 0.93)*	0.72 (0.58, 0.89)**	0.75 (0.61, 0.92)**	0.91 (0.77, 1.09)	0.94 (0.79, 1.11)
Region					
Northeast	Ref.	Ref.	Ref.	Ref.	Ref.
Midwest	0.66 (0.42, 1.02)	0.76 (0.55, 1.03)	0.49 (0.37, 0.65)***	0.93 (0.75, 1.17)	0.94 (0.75, 1.16)
South	0.80 (0.52, 1.24)	1.00 (0.74, 1.36)	0.59 (0.43, 0.80)**	1.23 (0.97, 1.57)	0.81 (0.68, 0.98)*
West	0.67 (0.43, 1.04)	0.62 (0.46, 0.85)**	0.45 (0.34, 0.60)***	1.47 (1.20, 1.79)***	0.83 (0.68, 1.02)
Household per capita income					

(continued)

Table 5.4 (continued)

	Preventive care				
	Blood pressure check within the previous 12 months (N = 14,643)	Cholesterol check within the previous 12 months (N = 14,341)	Routine checkup within the previous 12 months (N = 14,528)	Blood stool test within the previous 12 months (N = 13,820)	Breast exam within the previous 12 months (for women only) (N = 8025)
			OR (95% CI)		
0–9999	Ref.	Ref.	Ref.	Ref.	Ref.
10,000–24,999	1.33 (0.98, 1.81)	1.18 (0.97, 1.42)	1.20 (1.00, 1.44)*	1.07 (0.94, 1.23)	1.00 (0.86, 1.16)
25,000–49,999	1.45 (0.97, 2.16)	1.28 (1.01, 1.63)*	1.43 (1.12, 1.83)**	1.01 (0.85, 1.20)	1.26 (1.06, 1.50)*
50,000 or more	1.87 (1.18, 2.97)**	1.49 (1.09, 2.04)*	1.51 (1.13, 2.02)**	1.22 (0.97, 1.55)	1.48 (1.20, 1.83)***
Insurance coverage					
Uninsured	Ref.	Ref.	Ref.	Ref.	Ref.
Medicare only	1.63 (0.89, 2.98)	1.30 (0.73, 2.30)	1.79 (1.06, 3.03)*	1.35 (0.78, 2.32)	0.74 (0.42, 1.29)
Medicare and private	2.26 (1.17, 4.38)*	1.54 (0.86, 2.75)	2.02 (1.21, 3.37)**	1.19 (0.69, 2.06)	0.96 (0.55, 1.68)
Medicare and other public only	2.32 (1.28, 4.18)**	1.72 (0.95, 3.13)	1.77 (1.04, 3.03)*	1.35 (0.77, 2.36)	0.79 (0.44, 1.39)
No medicare and any public/private	0.95 (0.25, 3.68)	0.60 (0.17, 2.07)	1.19 (0.44, 3.23)	0.58 (0.18, 1.89)	1.29 (0.50, 3.34)
Need help with ADLs					
No	Ref.	Ref.	Ref.	Ref.	Ref.
Yes	1.65 (0.67, 4.07)	0.93 (0.65, 1.31)	0.86 (0.60, 1.23)	1.15 (0.88, 1.51)	0.93 (0.74, 1.17)
Need help with IADLs					
No	Ref.	Ref.	Ref.	Ref.	Ref.
Yes	1.00 (0.57, 1.78)	0.75 (0.57, 0.98)*	0.78 (0.59, 1.04)	1.07 (0.86, 1.34)	0.69 (0.57, 0.84)***
Number of chronic conditions	1.62 (1.46, 1.79)***	1.47 (1.40, 1.54)***	1.29 (1.24, 1.35)***	1.06 (1.03, 1.08)***	1.02 (0.99, 1.06)

(continued)

Table 5.4 (continued)

	Preventive care				
	Blood pressure check within the previous 12 months (N = 14,643)	Cholesterol check within the previous 12 months (N = 14,341)	Routine checkup within the previous 12 months (N = 14,528)	Blood stool test within the previous 12 months (N = 13,820)	Breast exam within the previous 12 months (for women only) (N = 8025)
			OR (95% CI)		
Provider's type					
Facility	Ref.	Ref.	Ref.	Ref.	Ref.
Person	0.98 (0.71, 1.36)	1.23 (1.00, 1.51)	1.23 (1.01, 1.49)*	1.00 (0.84, 1.20)	1.18 (1.01, 1.39)*
Person in facility Provider	1.43 (1.05, 1.94)*	1.17 (0.96, 1.43)	1.12 (0.95, 1.32)	0.88 (0.75, 1.04)	1.07 (0.93, 1.24)
Provider's location					
Office	Ref.	Ref.	Ref.	Ref.	Ref.
Hospital, not ER	0.69 (0.49, 0.97)*	1.02 (0.82, 1.28)	0.89 (0.74, 1.07)	1.22 (1.07, 1.39)**	1.02 (0.86, 1.21)
PCC attributes					
Whole person care					
No	Ref.	Ref.	Ref.	Ref.	Ref.
Yes	1.33 (0.99, 1.78)	2.45 (1.47, 4.08)**	1.75 (1.29, 2.38)***	1.20 (0.97, 1.48)	1.21 (0.99, 1.48)
Patient engagement and shared decision making					
No	Ref.	Ref.	Ref.	Ref.	Ref.
Yes	1.14 (1.01, 1.31)*	1.64 (1.25, 2.14)***	1.14 (1.01, 1.29)*	1.27 (1.16, 1.39)***	1.07 (0.97, 1.18)
Accessible care					
No	Ref.	Ref.	Ref.	Ref.	Ref.
Yes	0.99 (0.81, 1.21)	1.61 (1.08, 2.41)*	1.05 (0.87, 1.26)	1.16 (1.00, 1.36)	1.14 (0.99, 1.32)
Gender					
Male	–	–	–	Ref.	Ref.
Female	–	–	–	0.95 (0.86, 1.04)	1.02 (0.94, 1.11)

(continued)

Table 5.4 (continued)

	Preventive care				
	Blood pressure check within the previous 12 months (N = 14,643)	Cholesterol check within the previous 12 months (N = 14,341)	Routine checkup within the previous 12 months (N = 14,528)	Blood stool test within the previous 12 months (N = 13,820)	Breast exam within the previous 12 months (for women only) (N = 8025)
			OR (95% CI)		
Age	0.94 (0.93, 0.95)***	0.94 (0.92, 0.97)***	0.99 (0.98, 1.00)*	0.95 (0.94, 0.96)***	0.95 (0.94, 0.95)***
Race/ethnicity					
Non-Hispanic white only	Ref.	Ref.	Ref.	Ref.	Ref.
Hispanic	1.42 (1.13, 1.79)**	0.90 (0.59, 1.37)	0.90 (0.73, 1.12)	2.18 (1.88, 2.52)***	2.12 (1.83, 2.46)***
Non-Hispanic black only	1.38 (1.13, 1.68)**	0.91 (0.62, 1.33)	1.13 (0.91, 1.39)	1.35 (1.17, 1.55)***	1.41 (1.23, 1.61)***
Non-Hispanic Asian only	0.75 (0.59, 0.96)*	0.27 (0.17, 0.42)***	0.59 (0.44, 0.80)**	1.65 (1.28, 2.12)***	1.64 (1.32, 2.02)***
Non-Hispanic other race or multi-race	0.92 (0.49, 1.71)	1.56 (0.51, 4.77)	0.73 (0.45, 1.16)	1.11 (0.77, 1.59)	1.42 (0.98, 2.05)
Marital status					
Not married	Ref.	Ref.	Ref.	Ref.	Ref.
Married	1.46 (1.26, 1.69)***	1.00 (0.74, 1.37)	1.30 (1.10, 1.53)**	1.13 (1.02, 1.24)*	1.10 (1.00, 1.20)
Education					
No degree	Ref.	Ref.	Ref.	Ref.	Ref.
General Equivalency Diploma/high school diploma	1.39 (1.16, 1.66)***	1.12 (0.81, 1.55)	1.52 (1.27, 1.81)***	0.97 (0.87, 1.08)	1.10 (0.97, 1.24)
Bachelor's degree/some college/associate degree	1.47 (1.18, 1.84)**	1.90 (1.13, 3.20)*	1.48 (1.17, 1.89)**	0.95 (0.83, 1.08)	1.24 (1.07, 1.43)**
Advance degree	1.80 (1.32, 2.45)***	1.19 (0.71, 1.99)	1.43 (1.11, 1.85)**	0.92 (0.80, 1.07)	1.09 (0.92, 1.28)

(continued)

Table 5.4 (continued)

	Preventive care				
	Blood pressure check within the previous 12 months (N = 14,643)	Cholesterol check within the previous 12 months (N = 14,341)	Routine checkup within the previous 12 months (N = 14,528)	Blood stool test within the previous 12 months (N = 13,820)	Breast exam within the previous 12 months (for women only) (N = 8025)
			OR (95% CI)		
Employment status					
Not employed	Ref.	Ref.	Ref.	Ref.	Ref.
Employed	1.15 (0.89, 1.49)	0.74 (0.46, 1.19)	0.98 (0.82, 1.17)	0.99 (0.85, 1.14)	0.91 (0.79, 1.04)
Region					
Northeast	Ref.	Ref.	Ref.	Ref.	Ref.
Midwest	0.97 (0.76, 1.24)	0.92 (0.54, 1.59)	0.90 (0.71, 1.15)	0.88 (0.74, 1.05)	0.89 (0.74, 1.06)
South	0.98 (0.77, 1.25)	1.11 (0.75, 1.66)	0.99 (0.78, 1.25)	0.96 (0.83, 1.12)	0.95 (0.81, 1.12)
West	0.95 (0.74, 1.22)	1.20 (0.78, 1.85)	0.78 (0.59, 1.04)	0.87 (0.71, 1.06)	0.94 (0.79, 1.12)
Household per capita income					
0–9999	Ref.	Ref.	Ref.	Ref.	Ref.
10,000–24,999	1.07 (0.91, 1.26)	1.16 (0.87, 1.54)	1.00 (0.82, 1.20)	1.03 (0.90, 1.18)	1.03 (0.90, 1.19)
25,000–49,999	1.33 (1.10, 1.60)**	1.41 (0.94, 2.11)	1.29 (1.02, 1.61)*	1.06 (0.92, 1.22)	1.05 (0.91, 1.22)
50,000 or more	1.61 (1.23, 2.11)**	1.43 (0.85, 2.38)	1.36 (1.06, 1.74)*	1.17 (0.97, 1.40)	1.10 (0.90, 1.35)
Insurance coverage					
Uninsured	Ref.	Ref.	Ref.	Ref.	Ref.
Medicare only	2.46 (1.26, 4.80)**	1.70 (0.57, 5.01)	1.42 (0.83, 2.42)	1.27 (0.89, 1.80)	1.42 (1.00, 2.01)*
Medicare and private	3.28 (1.68, 6.41)**	2.94 (1.01, 8.59)*	1.63 (0.96, 2.77)	1.29 (0.91, 1.83)	1.50 (1.05, 2.15)*
Medicare and other public only	2.40 (1.22, 4.71)*	1.44 (0.49, 4.26)	1.45 (0.83, 2.53)	1.24 (0.85, 1.81)	1.40 (0.96, 2.06)

(continued)

Table 5.4 (continued)

	Preventive care				
	Blood pressure check within the previous 12 months (N = 14,643)	Cholesterol check within the previous 12 months (N = 14,341)	Routine checkup within the previous 12 months (N = 14,528)	Blood stool test within the previous 12 months (N = 13,820)	Breast exam within the previous 12 months (for women only) (N = 8025)
			OR (95% CI)		
No medicare and any public/private	1.33 (0.42, 4.26)	1.63 (0.20, 13.41)	0.73 (0.31, 1.72)	1.05 (0.44, 2.51)	1.22 (0.56, 2.65)
Need help with ADLs					
No	Ref.	Ref.	Ref.	Ref.	Ref.
Yes	0.63 (0.50, 0.80)***	0.81 (0.49, 1.32)	1.03 (0.76, 1.41)	0.92 (0.74, 1.14)	0.74 (0.58, 0.94)*
Need help with IADLs					
No	Ref.	Ref.	Ref.	Ref.	Ref.
Yes	0.67 (0.55, 0.82)***	0.61 (0.39, 0.95)*	0.71 (0.55, 0.92)*	0.86 (0.73, 1.00)	0.86 (0.73, 1.02)
Number of chronic conditions	1.05 (1.01, 1.09)**	1.11 (1.02, 1.19)*	1.04 (1.00 1.08)	1.32 (1.29, 1.36)***	1.26 (1.23, 1.30)***
Provider's type					
Facility	Ref.	Ref.	Ref.	Ref.	Ref.
Person	1.17 (0.99, 1.39)	0.91 (0.64, 1.31)	1.36 (1.13, 1.63)**	1.09 (0.95, 1.24)	1.08 (0.95, 1.23)
Person in facility Provider	1.07 (0.93, 1.23)	0.87 (0.61 1.26)	1.07 (0.89, 1.27)	1.02 (0.91, 1.16)	1.18 (1.04, 1.33)**
Provider's location					
Office	Ref.	Ref.	Ref.	Ref.	Ref.
Hospital, not ER	0.99 (0.80, 1.23)	0.91 (0.63, 1.32)	1.01 (0.85, 1.21)	1.02 (0.89, 1.16)	1.05 (0.91, 1.21)

$^*p < 0.05$, $^{**}p < 0.01$, $^{***}p < 0.001$

The analyses were weighted to reflect the complex survey design of MEPS

(95% CI: 1.01–1.31, $P < 0.05$) times more likely to get the mammogram within the previous 24 months, was 1.64 (95% CI: 1.25–2.14, $P < 0.001$) times more likely to receive Pap smear test, and was 1.14 (95% CI: 1.01–1.29, $P < 0.05$) times more likely to get the PSA test. It is worth noting that patient engagement attribute was also associated with higher odds in getting three gender-specific preventive screenings, which are breast exams, mammograms, Pap smear tests and the PSA tests.

With regard to the associations between enhanced access attribute and preventive care measures, the results showed that the attribute was significantly associated with higher odds in getting blood stool tests (OR: 1.36, 95% CI: 1.17–1.58) and Pap smear tests (OR: 1.61, 95% CI: 1.08–2.41) than the non-enhanced access group.

In terms of health education measures, the results showed that patient engagement attribute was significantly associated with higher odds in getting the healthy diet educations (OR:1.27, 95% CI: 1.16–1.39). No individual PCC attribute was found to be significantly associated with higher odds in getting the physical activity educations. The significant associations between other predictors and preventive care measures were also observed. The results were comparable and also confirmed the results associating PCC status with preventive screening and health education measures presented in the last section.

References

Greene, W. H. (2000). *Econometric analysis* (4th ed.). Prentice Hall.

Shi, L. (2012). The impact of primary care: A focused review. *Scientifica (Cairo), 2012*, 432892.

Tsai, J., Shi, L., Yu, W. L., & Lebrun, L. A. (2010). Usual source of care and the quality of medical care experiences: A cross-sectional survey of patients from a Taiwanese community. *Medical Care, 48*(7), 628–634.

Chapter 6
The Impact of Patient-Centered Care on Healthcare Outcomes

6.1 Introduction

This chapter presents the results for the second aims of the empirical study, which assessed the relationship between the receipt of PCC and chronic management, measured by the relationship between the receipt of PCC and chronic disease health outcomes, measured by the patient perceived health status and the incidence of adverse utilization events among older adults with chronic conditions.

The chapter has five sections. The chapter firstly describes the bivariate associations among the study variables. Then we present the results from the logistic regression models, which were used to examine the associations of PCC with health outcomes while individual sociodemographic and characteristics and system factors were controlled for. The chapter ends with an investigation of the relationships between each PCC attribute and health outcomes.

6.2 Bivariate Results

Table 4.3 shows the bivariate associations between the PCC status and the health outcome measures. Overall, the result of comparisons for two health status (physical and mental health) measures were significant at $P < 0.05$. The PCC patients were significantly more likely to perceive good health status and mental health status than the non-PCC patients. Similarly, the partial PCC group was also significantly associated with higher odds of perceiving good physical as well as mental health status. The differences in the two other health outcome measures (hospitalization and ER visits) were not statistically significant.

Between the two health status measures reported by all the respondents, a larger proportion of respondents reported good mental health status than good physical health status (89.9% vs. 78.9%). As for the measures for hospitalization and ER visits, around 16% of respondents reported that they were hospitalized in the past

H. Liang, *The Impact of Patient-Centered Care*,
https://doi.org/10.1007/978-981-16-3968-5_6

year, and approximately 18% of respondents reported that they had ER visits in the past year.

As for the comparison among the three groups, PCC and the partial PCC patients were significantly more likely to perceive good physical health status and mental health status. The differences between the PCC group and the non-PCC group for the two measures were 4.9 and 3.9%. However, the differences between the PCC group and the partial PCC group for the two measures were small (0.96 and 0.77%).

6.3 Multivariate Results

6.3.1 Multivariate Analysis: PCC Status Associated with Health Outcomes

Table 6.1 displays the multiple logistic regression results associating PCC with health outcome measures after control for individual predisposing, enabling, and need covariates as well as system covariates. The results relate the status of PCC (PCC vs. non-PCC, partial PCC vs. non-PCC) to the odds of four types of health outcome measures. Both the odds ratios and their 95% confidence intervals are presented. Similar to the findings from the bivariate analyses, even after control for individual and institutional characteristics, PCC and partial PCC patients were found to be more likely than the non-PCC patients to perceive good physical and mental health status, and PCC status was not found significantly associated with the hospitalization and ER visits.

As for the two perceived health status measures, both PCC status and partial PCC status were associated with higher odds in perceiving excellent/very good/good health and mental health status. Specifically, PCC group was 1.35 (95% CI: 1.18–1.56, $P <$ 0.001) times more likely than non-PCC group to perceive excellent/very good/good health, and was 1.46 (95% CI: 1.22–1.74, $P < 0.001$) times more likely than non-PCC group to perceive good mental health status. In contrast, the results showed PCC status was not significantly associated with the odds of getting hospitalization, and the PCC status was also not significantly associated with the odds of having ER visits.

Similarly, the partial PCC group was also associated with higher odds in perceiving excellent/very good/good health and mental health status than the non-PCC group. Specifically, the partial PCC group was 1.25 (95% CI: 1.10–1.43, $P < 0.01$) times more likely than non-PCC group to perceive excellent/very good/good health status, and was 1.33 (95% CI: 1.14–1.56, $P < 0.001$) times more likely than non-PCC group to perceive good mental health status. The results showed the partial PCC status was also not found significantly associated with the hospitalization and ER visits. Finally, with regard to the comparisons for magnitude of OR, the results showed that there were not much differences in magnitude of ORs between PCC and partial PCC.

The significant associations between other predictor variables of interest and preventive care measures were also observed. As for the predisposing factors, the results showed that female were more likely to perceive good mental health (OR: 1.19, 95% CI: 1.02–1.38). With the increase of age, we found one year older in age is associated with 2% higher odds of hospitalization (OR: 1.02, 95% CI: 1.01–1.03, $P < 0.001$) and 1% higher odds of having ER visits (OR: 1.01, 95% CI: 1.01–1.02, $P < 0.01$). As for the race/ethnicity, the results showed Hispanics were significantly associated with lower odds in perceiving good physical as well as mental health status. The negative associations were also found in the non-Hispanic Blacks. The non-Hispanic Asians was significantly associated with lower odds in perceiving good physical health status. The higher education level was also found associated with higher odds of perceiving good physical and mental health status. Similarly, patients who were employed were more likely to perceive good physical and mental health status. In terms of the predisposing factors, household per capital income level of USD 50,000 or above and level of USD 25,000–49,000 were significantly associated with higher odds in perceiving good health and mental health status than the level of USD 0–9999. Notably, the results showed that the insurance coverage status was not associated with all these four health outcome measures. Regarding the needs covariates, the need help with ADLs and IADLs were associated with lower odds of perceiving good health and mental health status, and were associated with higher odds of hospitalization and ER visits. Similarly, the increase of the number of chronic conditions was also associated with lower odds of perceiving good health and mental health status, and was associated with higher odds of hospitalization and ER visits. Finally, with regard to the system factors, the results showed that patients who visited person type providers (e.g. family physicians, primary care doctor in doctor's office rather than hospitals or ER) were associated with lower odds of having hospitalization, and patients whose provider's location was in hospitals were associated with lower odds of perceiving good health status.

6.3.2 Multivariate Analysis: PCC Attributes Associated with Health Outcomes

Table 6.2 displays the multiple logistic regression results associating PCC attributes with the four types of health outcomes after control for individual predisposing, enabling, and need covariates as well as system covariates. The results relate the attributes of PCC (whole person care vs. non-whole person care, patient engagement vs. non-patient engagement and enhanced access vs. non-enhanced access) to the odds of the health outcome measures. Both the odds ratios and their 95% confidence intervals are presented.

As for the two the health status measures, the whole person care attribute was not found significantly associated with either of the two measures. The patient engagement attribute was associated with higher odds in perceiving good mental health

Table 6.1 Multivariate analysis of correlates of health status and adverse utilization events

	Health status		Adverse event	
	Perceived health status: excellent/very good/good (N = 16,316)	Perceived mental good health status (N = 16,315)	Hospitalization (N = 16,404)	ER visits (N = 16,404)
	OR (95% CI)			
Patient-centered care				
Non-PCC	Ref.	Ref.	Ref.	Ref.
Partial-PCC	1.25 (1.10, 1.43)**	1.33 (1.14, 1.56)***	0.97 (0.85, 1.11)	0.99 (0.87, 1.12)
PCC	1.35 (1.18, 1.56)***	1.46 (1.22, 1.74)***	0.98 (0.84, 1.14)	0.91 (0.79, 1.05)
Gender				
Male	Ref.	Ref.	Ref.	Ref.
Female	1.07 (0.96, 1.19)	1.19 (1.02, 1.38)*	0.89 (0.79, 1.00)	1.02 (0.91, 1.13)
Age	1.01 (1.00, 1.02)*	1.00 (0.99, 1.01)	1.02 (1.01, 1.03)***	1.01 (1.01, 1.02)**
Race/ethnicity				
Non-Hispanic White only	Ref.	Ref.	Ref.	Ref.
Hispanic	0.56 (0.46, 0.67)***	0.71 (0.56, 0.89)**	0.89 (0.74, 1.06)	0.86 (0.71, 1.05)
Non-Hispanic Black only	0.72 (0.61, 0.86)***	0.75 (0.63, 0.90)**	1.01 (0.88, 1.15)	1.14 (0.99, 1.32)
Non-Hispanic Asian only	0.67 (0.53, 0.86)**	0.87 (0.64, 1.19)	0.76 (0.58, 1.01)	0.58 (0.44, 0.78)***
Non-Hispanic other race or multi-race	0.99 (0.69, 1.41)	0.60 (0.37, 0.99)*	1.03 (0.64, 1.66)	0.93 (0.56, 1.52)
Marital status				
Not married	Ref.	Ref.	Ref.	Ref.
Married	0.95 (0.83, 1.08)	1.11 (0.94, 1.31)	0.91 (0.81, 1.02)	0.88 (0.77, 0.99)*

(continued)

Table 6.1 (continued)

	Health status		Adverse event	
	Perceived health status: excellent/very good/good (N = 16,316)	Perceived mental good health status (N = 16,315)	Hospitalization (N = 16,404)	ER visits (N = 16,404)
	OR (95% CI)			
Education				
No degree	Ref.	Ref.	Ref.	Ref.
General equivalency diploma/high school diploma	1.52 (1.32, 1.76)***	1.42 (1.19, 1.69)***	0.90 (0.76, 1.06)	0.88 (0.76, 1.02)
Bachelor's degree/some college/associate degree	1.71 (1.40, 2.09)***	2.10 (1.65, 2.67)***	1.00 (0.84, 1.19)	0.88 (0.74, 1.04)
Advance degree	1.88 (1.51, 2.35)***	1.67 (1.23, 2.27)**	0.78 (0.63, 0.97)*	0.81 (0.66, 0.98)*
Employment status				
Not employed	Ref.	Ref.	Ref.	Ref.
Employed	1.43 (1.19, 1.73)***	1.56 (1.19, 2.06)**	1.03 (0.87, 1.22)	0.90 (0.76, 1.05)
Region				
Northeast	Ref.	Ref.	Ref.	Ref.
Midwest	1.11 (0.93, 1.33)	1.15 (0.89, 1.49)	0.97 (0.81, 1.16)	0.91 (0.76, 1.09)
South	0.90 (0.76, 1.06)	0.97 (0.77, 1.22)	0.88 (0.76, 1.02)	0.77 (0.66, 0.90)**
West	1.06 (0.87, 1.30)	1.00 (0.78, 1.29)	0.79 (0.66, 0.93)**	0.85 (0.71, 1.01)
Household per capita income				
0–9999	Ref.	Ref.	Ref.	Ref.
10,000–24,999	1.25 (1.09, 1.42)**	1.05 (0.88, 1.26)	0.96 (0.81, 1.12)	0.97 (0.84, 1.13)

(continued)

Table 6.1 (continued)

	Health status		Adverse event	
	Perceived health status: excellent/very good/good (N = 16,316)	Perceived mental good health status (N = 16,315)	Hospitalization (N = 16,404)	ER visits (N = 16,404)
	OR (95% CI)			
25,000–49,999	1.51 (1.29, 1.77)***	1.36 (1.05, 1.75)*	0.79 (0.67, 0.93)**	0.90 (0.74, 1.09)
50,000 or more	1.89 (1.49, 2.39)***	2.44 (1.74, 3.43)***	0.84 (0.67, 1.05)	0.97 (0.78, 1.22)
Insurance coverage				
Uninsured	Ref.	Ref.	Ref.	Ref.
Medicare only	1.36 (0.77, 2.40)	1.18 (0.54, 2.56)	1.47 (0.69, 3.14)	1.44 (0.70, 2.98)
Medicare and private	1.52 (0.86, 2.70)	1.13 (0.52, 2.44)	1.68 (0.79, 3.55)	1.57 (0.76, 3.25)
Medicare and other public only	1.03 (0.59, 1.81)	1.03 (0.47, 2.26)	1.34 (0.63, 2.85)	1.36 (0.65, 2.84)
No medicare and any public/private	1.68 (0.52, 5.42)	1.83 (0.43, 7.85)	1.04 (0.27, 3.95)	1.68 (0.60, 4.67)
Need help with ADLs				
No	Ref.	Ref.	Ref.	Ref.
Yes	0.39 (0.31, 0.48)***	0.58 (0.46, 0.73)***	1.90 (1.54, 2.34)***	1.93 (1.53, 2.43)***
Need help with IADLs				
No	Ref.	Ref.	Ref.	Ref.
Yes	0.38 (0.32, 0.46)***	0.26 (0.21, 0.31)***	1.58 (1.32, 1.90)***	1.52 (1.25, 1.84)***
Number of chronic conditions	0.71 (0.68, 0.73)***	0.88 (0.85, 0.91)***	1.25 (1.22, 1.29)***	1.21 (1.18 1.25)***
Provider's type				

(continued)

Table 6.1 (continued)

	Health status		Adverse event	
	Perceived health status: excellent/very good/good (N = 16,316)	Perceived mental good health status (N = 16,315)	Hospitalization (N = 16,404)	ER visits (N = 16,404)
	OR (95% CI)			
Facility	Ref.	Ref.	Ref.	Ref.
Person	1.07 (0.92, 1.23)	0.89 (0.75, 1.04)	0.83 (0.70, 0.98)*	0.91 (0.79, 1.04)
Person in facility provider	1.14 (0.99, 1.32)	1.01 (0.83, 1.24)	1.04 (0.90, 1.20)	1.13 (1.00, 1.27)
Provider's location				
Office	Ref.	Ref.	Ref.	Ref.
Hospital, not ER	0.84 (0.73, 0.98)*	0.88 (0.75, 1.04)	0.97 (0.83, 1.13)	1.09 (0.97, 1.22)

$*p < 0.05$, $**p < 0.01$, $***p < 0.001$
The analyses were weighted to reflect the complex survey design of MEPS

status. Specifically, the patient who got patient engagement was 1.28 (95% CI: 1.11–1.47, $P < 0.01$) times more likely to perceive good mental health status than the patient who did not get patient engagement.

With regard to the associations between enhanced access attribute and perceived health status measures, the results showed that the attribute was significantly associated with higher odds in perceiving excellent/very good/good health status (OR: 1.18, 95% CI: 1.01–1.38) than the non-enhanced access group.

In terms of measures for the hospitalization and ER visits, the results showed that the enhanced access attribute was significantly associated with lower odds in having ER visits (OR:0.84, 95% CI: 0.73–0.96). No individual PCC attribute was found to be significantly associated with lower odds in hospitalization. The significant associations between other predictors and health outcome measures were also observed. The results were comparable with the results associating PCC status with health outcome measures presented in the last sections (Table 6.3).

Table 6.2 Multivariate analysis of correlates of PCC attributes with health status and adverse event

	Health status		Adverse event	
	Perceived health status: excellent/very good/good (N = 14,733)	Perceived good mental health status (N = 14,737)	Hospitalization (N = 14,744)	ER visits (N = 14,744)
	OR (95% CI)			
PCC attributes				
Whole person care				
No	Ref.	Ref.	Ref.	Ref.
Yes	1.20 (0.95, 1.52)	1.19 (0.85, 1.66)	0.74 (0.54, 1.01)	0.88 (0.66, 1.16)
Patient engagement and shared decision making				
No	Ref.	Ref.	Ref.	Ref.
Yes	1.10 (0.99, 1.23)	1.28 (1.11, 1.47)**	1.08 (0.96, 1.22)	0.99 (0.89, 1.11)
Accessible care				
No	Ref.	Ref.	Ref.	Ref.
Yes	1.18 (1.01, 1.38)*	1.00 (0.80, 1.24)	0.90 (0.78, 1.03)	0.84 (0.73, 0.96)**
Gender				
Male	Ref.	Ref.	Ref.	Ref.
Female	1.07 (0.96, 1.20)	1.20 (1.03, 1.39)*	0.89 (0.79, 1.00)	1.01 (0.91, 1.13)
Age	1.01 (1.00, 1.02)*	1.00 (0.99, 1.01)	1.02 (1.01, 1.03)***	1.01 (1.00, 1.02)*
Race/ethnicity				
Non-Hispanic White only	Ref.	Ref.	Ref.	Ref.
Hispanic	0.56 (0.46, 0.68)***	0.72 (0.57, 0.91)**	0.89 (0.74, 1.06)	0.86 (0.71, 1.04)
Non-Hispanic Black only	0.73 (0.61, 0.86)***	0.76 (0.64, 0.91)**	1.01 (0.88, 1.16)	1.15 (0.99, 1.32)
Non-Hispanic Asian only	0.68 (0.53, 0.86)**	0.90 (0.66, 1.22)	0.78 (0.59, 1.03)	0.59 (0.44, 0.79)**

(continued)

Table 6.2 (continued)

	Health status		Adverse event	
	Perceived health status: excellent/very good/good (N = 14,733)	Perceived good mental health status (N = 14,737)	Hospitalization (N = 14,744)	ER visits (N = 14,744)
	OR (95% CI)			
Non-Hispanic other race or multi-race	0.97 (0.68, 1.39)	0.59 (0.36, 0.97)*	1.02 (0.63, 1.65)	0.92 (0.56, 1.52)
Marital status				
Not married	Ref.	Ref.	Ref.	Ref.
Married	0.95 (0.83, 1.09)	1.11 (0.93, 1.31)	0.91 (0.81, 1.02)	0.88 (0.77, 0.99)*
Education				
No degree	Ref.	Ref.	Ref.	Ref.
General equivalency diploma/high school diploma	1.52 (1.32, 1.76)***	1.42 (1.19, 1.69)***	0.90 (0.76, 1.06)	0.88 (0.76, 1.01)
Bachelor's degree/some college/associate degree	1.73 (1.41, 2.11)***	2.11 (1.66, 2.69)***	1.00 (0.84, 1.19)	0.87 (0.74, 1.03)
Advance degree	1.89 (1.52, 2.36)***	1.66 (1.22, 2.26)**	0.78 (0.63, 0.97)*	0.80 (0.66, 0.98)*
Employment status				
Not employed	Ref.	Ref.	Ref.	Ref.
Employed	1.44 (1.20, 1.73)***	1.57 (1.19, 2.06)**	1.03 (0.87, 1.22)	0.90 (0.76, 1.05)
Region				
Northeast	Ref.	Ref.	Ref.	Ref.
Midwest	1.11 (0.93, 1.33)	1.15 (0.89, 1.49)	0.97 (0.81, 1.16)	0.91 (0.76, 1.09)
South	0.90 (0.77, 1.06)	0.96 (0.76, 1.21)	0.87 (0.75, 1.01)	0.77 (0.66, 0.90)**

(continued)

Table 6.2 (continued)

	Health status		Adverse event	
	Perceived health status: excellent/very good/good (N = 14,733)	Perceived good mental health status (N = 14,737)	Hospitalization (N = 14,744)	ER visits (N = 14,744)
	OR (95% CI)			
West	1.05 (0.86, 1.28)	0.99 (0.77, 1.27)	0.78 (0.66, 0.93)**	0.85 (0.71, 1.01)
Household per capita income				
0–9999	Ref.	Ref.	Ref.	Ref.
10,000–24,999	1.25 (1.09, 1.42)**	1.05 (0.88, 1.26)	0.95 (0.81, 1.12)	0.97 (0.84, 1.12)
25,000–49,999	1.51 (1.29, 1.76)***	1.36 (1.05, 1.75)*	0.79 (0.67, 0.93)**	0.90 (0.74, 1.09)
50,000 or more	1.88 (1.49, 2.38)***	2.45 (1.75, 3.42)***	0.83 (0.66, 1.05)	0.97 (0.78, 1.22)
Insurance coverage				
Uninsured	Ref.	Ref.	Ref.	Ref.
Medicare only	1.35 (0.77, 2.38)	1.17 (0.54, 2.55)	1.47 (0.70, 3.13)	1.43 (0.69, 2.94)
Medicare and private	1.52 (0.86, 2.69)	1.13 (0.52, 2.45)	1.68 (0.80, 3.54)	1.56 (0.76, 3.20)
Medicare and other public only	1.02 (0.58, 1.79)	1.02 (0.46, 2.25)	1.34 (0.64, 2.84)	1.35 (0.65, 2.81)
No medicare and any public/private	1.68 (0.51, 5.48)	1.84 (0.43, 7.92)	1.05 (0.28, 3.99)	1.67 (0.60, 4.62)
Need help with ADLs				
No	Ref.	Ref.	Ref.	Ref.
Yes	0.38 (0.31, 0.48)***	0.59 (0.47, 0.74)***	1.90 (1.54, 2.35)***	1.93 (1.53, 2.44)

(continued)

Table 6.2 (continued)

	Health status		Adverse event	
	Perceived health status: excellent/very good/good (N = 14,733)	Perceived good mental health status (N = 14,737)	Hospitalization (N = 14,744)	ER visits (N = 14,744)
	OR (95% CI)			
Need help with IADLs				
No	Ref.	Ref.	Ref.	Ref.
Yes	0.38 (0.32, 0.46)***	0.25 (0.21, 0.31)***	1.59 (1.33, 1.91)***	1.52 (1.25, 1.84)
Number of chronic conditions	0.71 (0.69, 0.73)***	0.88 (0.85, 0.91)***	1.25 (1.21, 1.29)***	1.21 (1.18, 1.25)
Provider's type				
Facility	Ref.	Ref.	Ref.	Ref.
Person	1.08 (0.93, 1.24)	0.88 (0.75, 1.03)	0.82 (0.69, 0.97)*	0.89 (0.78, 1.02)
Person in facility provider	1.14 (0.98, 1.33)	1.00 (0.81, 1.22)	1.03 (0.89, 1.19)	1.11 (0.99, 1.26)
Provider's location				
Office	Ref.	Ref.	Ref.	Ref.
Hospital, not ER	0.84 (0.72, 0.97)*	0.88 (0.75, 1.03)	0.97 (0.84, 1.13)	1.09 (0.97, 1.23)

*$p < 0.05$, **$p < 0.01$, ***$p < 0.001$

The analyses were weighted to reflect the complex survey design of MEPS

Table 6.3 Health status and adverse events: comparisons between patient-centered care patients and non patient-centered care patients

	Total	Patient-centered care	Partial patient-centered care	Non-patient-centered care	*P* value
	% (95% CI)				
Sample size (unweighted)	16,654	5963	6973	3718	
Weighted population (1000)	181,599.05	64,748.36	76,168.68	40,682.01	
Perceived health status: excellent/very good/good (N = 16,316)	78.89 (77.82, 79.92)	80.39 (79.01, 81.71)	79.43 (78.03, 80.76)	75.50 (73.53, 77.36)	<0.001
Perceived good mental health status (N = 16,315)	89.94 (89.23, 90.60)	91.14 (90.09, 92.09)	90.37 (89.41, 91.26)	87.20 (85.72, 88.54)	<0.001
Hospitalization (N = 16,404)	16.16 (15.41, 16.94)	16.09 (14.90, 17.35)	15.94 (14.94, 17.00)	16.68 (15.18, 18.30)	0.71
ER visits (N = 16,404)	18.13 (17.37, 18.93)	17.30 (16.20, 18.47)	18.32 (17.22, 19.47)	19.10 (17.52, 20.80)	0.16

The actual sample and population size vary because of missing or inapplicable values for different measures. The analyses were weighted to reflect the complex survey design of MEPS

Chapter 7
The Patient-Centered Care on Cancer Prevention and Treatment

7.1 Introduction

Optimal cancer care entails the coordination among multiple providers, continued follow-up and surveillance over time. The patient-centered care brings opportunities to improve the delivery of cancer care. The adoption of patient-centered oncology care (PCOC) is in its infancy. Evidence synthesis on the model's effectiveness is scant. This chapter presents a systemic review and meta-analysis on associations of PCOC with cancer patients' adverse healthcare utilization, cost, patient satisfaction and quality of care. The chapter was guided by the Preferred Reporting Items for Systematic Reviews and Meta-Analyses (PRISMA) framework. Quality appraisal was performed using Downs and Black's quality checklist. Study-level effect sizes of adverse healthcare utilization were computed using Cohen's D and summarized using forest plots. Funnel plots were constructed to examine publication bias.

Of 334 studies that were reviewed, ten met eligibility criteria and were included into the final analysis. Many included studies implemented almost all six of patient-centered care core attributes, plus three additional attributes that specifically addressed cancer patients' needs, including triage pathways, standardized and evidence-based symptom management, as well as support patient navigation. PCOC patients had lower utilization of inpatient care (standardized means difference [SMD] $= -0.027$, $P = 0.049$). Overall positive effect of PCOC on emergency department use was small and not significant (SMD $= -0.023$, $P = 0.103$). In terms of cost and quality of care, our narrative summaries showed an overall positive direction, though we found limitations in individual study quality that precluded a meta-analysis.

The results showed that it is possible to utilize patient-centered model to support best-practice of cancer care. Early evidence shows that the PCOC model has potential to improve healthcare utilization, cost and quality of care, but limited numbers of included articles and heterogeneity of those studies implied that more rigorous research is expected to further investigate the model's effects.

H. Liang, *The Impact of Patient-Centered Care*,
https://doi.org/10.1007/978-981-16-3968-5_7

7.2 The Patient-Centered Oncology Care

Cancer has a major impact on society worldwide and is the second leading cause of death in the United States. Currently, the number of patient living with a cancer diagnosis is projected to increase, it is mainly due to the increase in the incidence of cancer (National Cancer Institute, 2018). The US has 15.5 million individuals living with a cancer diagnosis, a number projected to reach 19 million by 2024 (American Cancer Society, 2017). In 2017, it was estimated that 1,688,780 new cancer cases were diagnosed and 600,920 people died of cancer in the US (American Cancer Society, 2017). All these newly diagnosed cancer patients demand medical care at every stage of their cancer experiences. The Institute of Medicine (IOM)'s report identified six major phases in the cancer care continuum: prevention, early detection, diagnosis, treatment, survivorship, and end-of-life care (Hewitt et al., 2005). The greater intensity of health care service use by cancer patients trigger increasing health care cost, resulting in a greater overall burden of cancer. It is estimated that the direct medical costs for cancer in the US in 2014 were $87.8 billion (American Cancer Society, 2017). Besides mounting cancer incidence rates, an increasing cost of medications and technologies, the excessive utilization of inpatient and emergency services coupled with fragmented care delivery are all contributing to the overall burden of cancer care (Ahmed et al., 2015).

Optimal and cost-effective cancer care entails the coordination of efforts from multiple providers, the use of several procedures and medications, coupled with continued follow-up and surveillance over time. Moreover, many health conditions are associated with cancer. For example, people age 65 and older are more likely to have one or more chronic health problems in addition to living with cancer at all stages, which include high blood pressure, heart disease, diabetes, and arthritis, etc. (National Cancer Institute, 2016). With increased disease burden, it requires innovative patient-management model and alternative payment reforms (Edwards et al., 2014; Wilper et al., 2008). Placing emphasis on team-based care, care coordination, patient-centered orientation, enhanced access to care, and quality improvement (Arend et al., 2012), the patient-centered medical home (PCMH) model brings opportunities to evolve and improve the delivery of cancer care. The PCMH has emerged as a solution to fragmented care delivery, which was developed to create a strong physician–patient relationship that results in more personal, coordinated, effective, and efficient care (National Committee for Quality Assurance [NCQA], 2011). PCMHs models have been applied broadly in different clinical settings and to different types of patients and settings, including in community health centers, chronic disease patients, and low-income or medically underserved populations (Hoff et al., 2012; Liang et al., 2017; Shi et al., 2017). A number of studies and literature reviews have shown that PCMHs are effective in improving patients' outcomes, quality of care as well as reducing costs among general populations (Arend et al., 2012; Hoff et al., 2012; Jackson et al., 2013; Reibling, 2016). Two recent systematic reviews also concluded that PCMH adoption was effective among specific population sub-groups, such as low-income and diabetic patients (McManus, 2017; van den Berk-Clark et al., 2017).

As health reform efforts to improve quality and experience of care move forward, PCMH models are incorporated into more health care settings, preferring value over volume and redesigning the entire health care delivery system (Huang & Rosenthal, 2014). For example, building on the success of the PCMH, the NCQA announced a Patient-Centered Specialty Practice (PCSP) recognition program in 2013, which is a practice-based evaluation for clinicians who provide care in non-primary care specialties. It puts patients first, requires providers to organize care around patients—across all clinicians seen by a patient—and to include patients in planning care and as partners in managing conditions (NCQA, 2013). The PCSP program is valuable for building delivery system reforms that go beyond primary care, while strengthening and clarifying the roles of both primary care and specialty practices (NCQA, 2013). Envisioning a patient-centered, triage pathway for the patients, potential advantages of PCSP models become clear. A practice with the PCSP recognition would have mechanisms in place to provide patients prompt access for clinical consultations. Primary care providers are involved at each step in the patient's care, and streamlined referrals could be well-coordinated. Patients would have seen a specialist in a timely manner and can focus more on their health needs rather than navigating the health system. Redundant testing and unnecessary medical procedures can be avoided (NCQA, 2013). One example of such specialty practices is the adoption of patient-centered models in cancer treatment. The NCQA, in conjunction with the American Society of Clinical Oncology (ASCO), the RAND Corporation, National Coalition for Cancer Survivorship, and Independence Blue Cross, was piloting a patient-centered oncology care (PCOC) model within a Patient-Centered Outcomes Research Institute–funded project in southeastern Pennsylvania. Early evidence showed these oncology practices in Pennsylvania successfully demonstrated that implementation of a PCSP-like model in cancer care. These efforts have the potential to bend the cost curve while also improving quality of care and patient satisfaction (Page et al., 2015).

One of the greatest challenges in cancer care is avoiding emergency department (ED) visits and unplanned hospitalizations during treatment and survivorship (American Cancer Society, 2013). Moreover, managing cost and quality for oncology care is also challenging. Innovative patient-management models in oncology based on PCMH principles, coupled with alternative payments, such as bundled payment and pay-for-performance, showed evidence of effectiveness, with bended curve of cost, improved quality of care and enhanced patient outcomes (Collins et al., 2010; Eagle & Sprandio, 2012; Page et al., 2015). The PCOC model represents a logical platform on which to build a more comprehensive value-oriented, evidence-based cancer care delivery system.

The adoption of PCOC is in its infancy. Importantly, systematic review and evidence synthesis on the model's effectiveness is scant. Our present study will address this knowledge gap and is particularly timely given the recent launch of the Centers for Medicare and Medicaid Services (CMS) Oncology Care Model. The latter is a new payment and delivery model incorporating elements of care coordination, navigation, and national treatment guidelines for cancer care (CMS, 2016a, 2016b). Evidence from our study can inform the implementation of PCOC.

7.3 Evidence Synthesis

Search Strategy

Comprehensive search strategies were applied during the electronic search of four databases: PubMed, Cochrane Library, EMBASE, and Google Scholar. The year of publication was set from January 1st, 2007 to May 31st, 2018. Our searching key words and MeSH terms include: "patient-centered medical home", "medical home", "patient-centered care (MeSH term)", "oncology medical home", "whole person orientation", "patient-focused care", and "delivery of health care, integrated" (MeSH term). We also filtered for "cancer", "neoplasms" (MeSH term) and "oncology".

Definition of PCOC and Conceptual Framework

In 2007, the major primary care physician associations endorsed the concept and Joint Principles of the PCMH, which was best described as a model or philosophy of care that is patient-centered, comprehensive, team-based, coordinated, accessible, and focused on quality and safety (Patient-Centered Primary Care Collaborative, 2012). In 2011, the NCQA proposed the PCMH standards which include 6 core principles: (1) enhance access and continuity, (2) use data for population management, (3) care management, (4) support self-care process, (5) referral tracking and follow-up and (6) implement continuous quality improvement (NCQA, 2011). In this study, we adopted the above definition and principles, and constructed a conceptual framework to guide this study (Fig. 7.1). The framework represents a heuristic for understanding of the demonstrated linkages between PCOC interventions and specific health care outcomes. As presented in Fig. 7.1, the conceptual framework for PCOC is centered around six PCMH dimensional constructs and three oncology-specific dimensional constructs that may lead to expected outcomes (Patient-Centered Primary Care Collaborative, 2012; Wender & Altshuler, 2009). For example, the dimension of identifying and managing patient population may help to facilitate care of less activated patients, such as assessing and documenting patient risk factors, and therefore identifying patients for proactive reminders. The other mechanism is that PCOC supports patients by establishing relationships with providers involved in their care during active treatment and connecting patients with community and financial resources (Arend et al., 2012; Jackson et al., 2013). Strong physician–patient relationships make care more coordinated, effective, and efficient (Hoff et al., 2012; Reibling, 2016). Moreover, under PCOC model, practices systematically record patient information for patient populations and uses it to coordinate patient care (NCQA, 2011).

In terms of three additional components related to oncology care, they were extracted based on the synthesized evidence from CMS on key drivers for improving oncology care (CMS, 2017). The three additional components extend current conceptualization of PCMH, and particularly target oncology outcomes and the delivery of quality and value in cancer care (ASCO, 2014; CMS, 2017). In terms of triage pathway, the PCOC practices may identify and implement pathways for disease

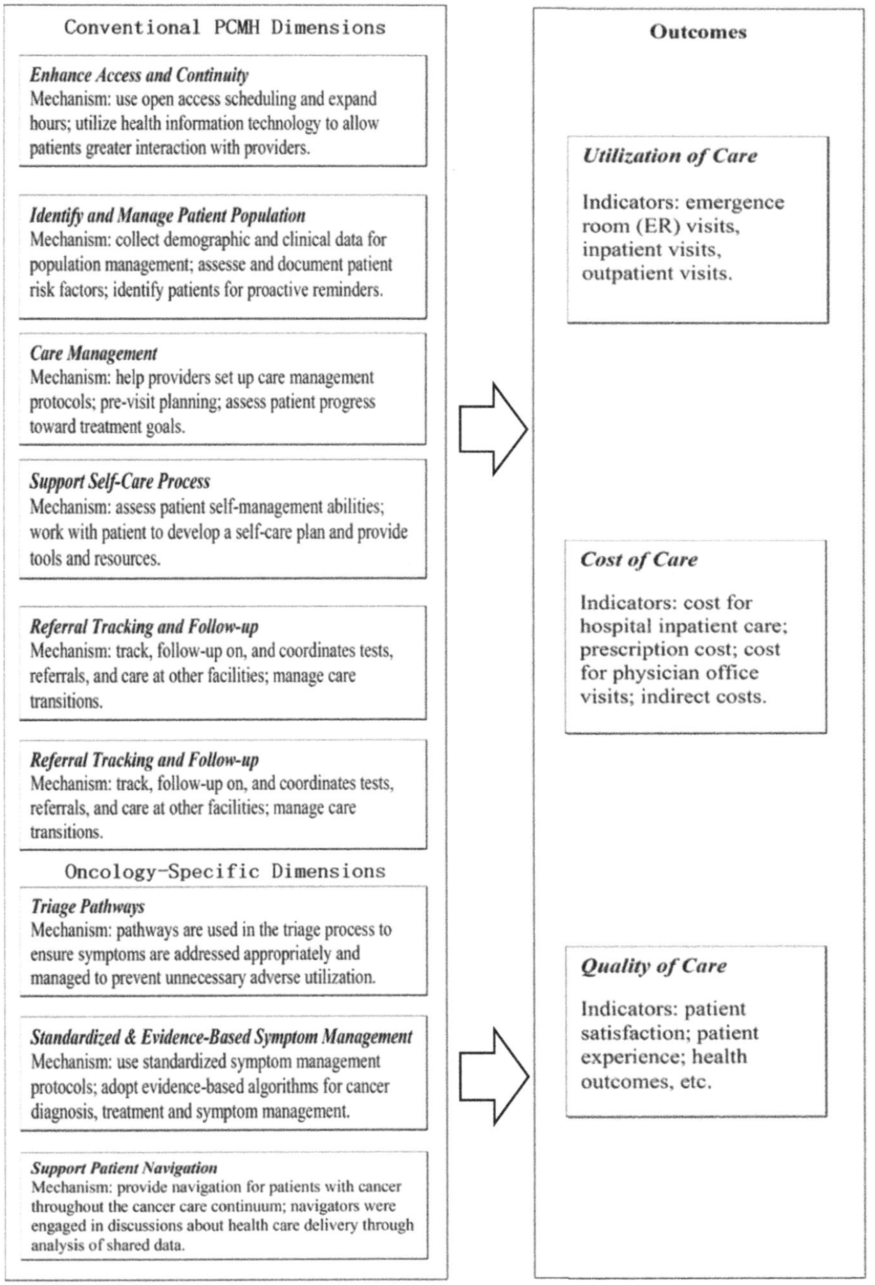

Fig. 7.1 Conceptual framework for patient-centered oncology care. *Note* The framework is adapted from the Joint Principles of the PCMH (PCPPC, 2012), and Wender and Altshuler (2009)

management that address common side effects experienced by its patient population. Besides, pathways are used in the triage process to ensure health problems are addressed appropriately and proactively managed to prevent unnecessary ER visits and impatient utilization (Eagle & Sprandio, 2012; Sprandio, 2010). For standardized and evidence-based symptom management, the PCOC practices may adopt evidence-based algorithms or tools for appropriate diagnosis, treatment and symptom management. These tools can be electronic or manual, but should be used systematically to ensure a standardized approach to providing evidence-based cancer care (Kuntz et al., 2014; Page et al., 2015). With respect to patient navigation support, it helps remove any roadblocks to treatment, so that patients and their families are able to find and make use of the various resources, treatment services, and support services that they need to receive the best cancer treatment possible (Kohler et al., 2015; Wheeler et al., 2013). If these above dimensions work in the intended manner, then expected outcomes would include lower utilization of high-cost care, cost savings and better quality of care (Patient-Centered Primary Care Collaborative, 2012; Rosenthal, 2008; Wender & Altshuler, 2009).

Study Selection

Initial records were identified from four electronic databases. Figure 7.2 outlines the screening process. Using the reference management software Endnote 8.0, duplicates were excluded automatically. Next, two independent investigators read the title and abstract of the related articles and assessed them according to the following selection criteria: (1) the intervention is a PCMH model that meets the six PCMH dimensional constructs in the conceptual framework; (2) research design is randomized controlled trial, cohort study, case control study, or case series; (3) stages of cancer care include any stages; (4) intervention is conducted at any types of setting (such as primary care and specialists); (5) conducted in the United States.

Articles that met these criteria or could not be clearly identified through the title and abstract screening would be kept for the next screening stage. Any disagreements were resolved through discussion between the two investigators (HL and LT). Through this stage, studies were excluded, remaining studies to full-text screening. Two investigators read the full texts of the remaining articles to assess them according to the following inclusion criteria: (1) the model meet the core principles of the PCMH, (2) the participants are cancer patients, (3) the purpose or outcomes is focused on healthcare utilization, cost, patient satisfaction and quality of care. Finally, eligible articles were finalized and data were extracted. We extracted data on author, publication year, study design, participants, description of the intervention, types of outcome, results and quality index. Table 7.1 describes the above characteristics of each articles.

Quality Assessment

Two investigators independently assessed the quality of the included studies based on the Downs and Blacks Checklists. The checklists contain a total of 27 items in 5 sections. Each item is given based on the answer to a detailed score, the higher the final score, the higher the quality of the literature, with an overall score of 33. Accordingly,

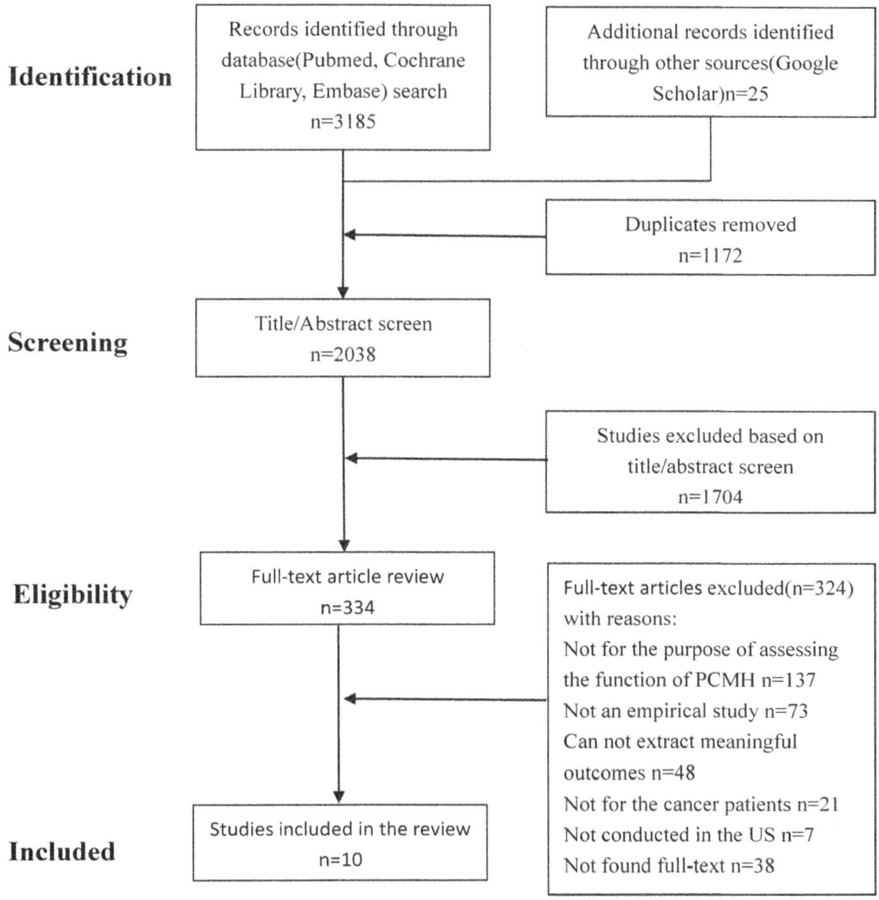

Fig. 7.2 Screening process for the eligible studies

the quality of the studies is divided into three levels based on the final score: low quality (1–11), medium quality (12–22), high quality (23–33). Disagreements about the final score were solved by two investigators through consultation.

Data Synthesis and Analysis

All analyses were conducted using Stata 12.0 (StataCorp, 2011). We extracted the outcomes into three main categories: (1) the utilization of care (emergence room [ER] visits, inpatient visits, and outpatient visits); (2) cost of care; (3) the quality of care and patient satisfaction. Study-level effect sizes of adverse healthcare utilization were computed using Cohen's *D* with the Bessel's correction and summarized using forest plots. We used a random effects model. The heterogeneity in the meta-analysis was assessed using Cochran Q test and I^2 statistics. Funnel plots and Egger's test were

Table 7.1 Study characteristics

Author, year	Study design	Data and analysis	Intervention group	Comparison group	Outcomes	Key findings	Quality appraisal
Sullivan et al. (2018)	Cohort study	Cancer registry data and Medicaid claims data from January, 2007 to June, 2013	15,369 cancer patients enrolled in the integrated care system	6491 cancer patients from the same cohort but never in the integrated care system	Enrollment, mean days	Increased hospice enrollment (OR = 1.07; $P < 0.001$), decreased time to enroll hospice (HR = 1.04; $P < 0.001$)	Medium (score 12)
Colligan et al. (2017a)	Cohort study	Medicare claim data from July 1, 2013 through June 30, 2015	3322 cancer patients from oncology medical home	3322 similar comparators	Emergency department (ER) visits, hospitalization, health care costs	Fewer ED visits (D = −0.007; $P < 0.01$), more hospitalizations (D = −0.013), decreased spending (D = −$675, $P < 0.01$)	High (score 25)
Colligan et al. (2017b)	Cohort study	Medicare claims data from June 2012 to December 2015	1244 cancer patients from oncology medical homes	1244 similar comparators	ER visits, hospitalization, health care costs	Fewer hospitalizations (D = −0.057), decreased costs (D = −$3346, $P < 0.01$)	Medium (score 18)
Kohler et al. (2015)	Cohort study	Medical claims linked to cancer registry records from 2003 to 2007	381 breast cancer women from a patient-centered medical home (PCMH)	377 women not enrolled in the PCMH	ER visits, hospitalizations, outpatient visits, and Medicaid expenditure	Increased outpatient service use (marginal effect = 0.5252, $P <$ 0.001), increased average expenditures (marginal effect = $429, $P < 0.1$)	High (score 23)

(continued)

Table 7.1 (continued)

Author, year	Study design	Data and analysis	Intervention group	Comparison group	Outcomes	Key findings	Quality appraisal
Waters et al. (2015)	Descriptive study	Medial claims at 2012 and 2014	16,353 cancer patients who enrolled in oncology medical homes	Historical comparison with their own data	Patient satisfaction, the volume of triage call	Rapid increase in triage call volume, patient satisfaction always above 90%	Medium (score 14)
Harper et al. (2015)	Descriptive study	Patient survey at 2012	52 cancer patients who received patient-centered oncology care	NA	Patient satisfaction	Patients rated the quality of patient-centered oncology care highly (mean 4.7, range [1 = poor to 5 = excellent]), and felt comfortable with their plan of care (mean 1.63, range [1 = extremely comfortable to 5 = not at all comfortable])	Medium (score 18)
Goyal et al. (2014)	Cohort study	Cancer registry data and Medicaid claims data from January 1, 2003 to December 31, 2007	308 women enrolled in a medical home program	262 women from the same cohort but never enrolled in the medical home program	ER visits, hospitalization and outpatient visits	Fewer inpatient admissions (marginal effect = −0.1421 (−0.280 to −0.004))	High (score 23)

(continued)

Table 7.1 (continued)

Author, year	Study design	Data and analysis	Intervention group	Comparison group	Outcomes	Key findings	Quality appraisal
Kuntz et al. (2014)	Descriptive study	Medical claims and patient survey at 2013	85 cancer patients from four practices participated a oncology medical home demonstration project	The averages from the previous 3 years at the four participating practices	ER visits, hospitalizations, cost savings, compliance with guidelines	Cost savings of $550 per patient	Medium (score 16)
Wheeler et al. (2013)	Cohort study	Cancer registry and Medicaid claims from 2003 to 2007	Half of 840 women breast cancer patients enrolled in a medical home program	The rest of women from the same cohort who did not enrolled in medical home program	Receipt of follow-up mammogram and physical examinations/history taking	The medical home enrollment was significantly positively associated with receipt of follow-up mammogram (marginal effect = 0.012, $P = 0.021$)	Medium (score 19)
Sprandio (2010)	Descriptive study	Medical records from 2005 to 2009	5606 cancer patients who enrolled in an oncology PCMH model	Historical comparison with their own data	Hospitalizations, ER visits	ER utilization rates decreased from 2 per person to 1 per person, patient had 16% reduction in hospital admissions	Medium (score 12)

constructed to examine publication bias. A funnel plot is a simple scatter plot of the intervention effect estimates from individual studies against measure of each study's size or precision. Using Egger's test, *P* value was calculated by a linear regression of intervention effect estimate against its standard error, weighted by the inverse of the variance of the intervention effect estimate (Egger et al., 1997). Other outcomes such as quality of care and patient satisfaction, cost of care and outpatient visits for reviews where the nature of data were diverse and not feasible to be extracted for quantitative syntheses. We summarized characteristics of studies in Table 7.1 and provide narrative descriptions for each included study. The Preferred Reporting Items for Systematic Reviews and Meta-Analyses (PRISMA) framework guided the conduct and reporting of this study (Moher et al., 2009).

7.4 Evidence on the Patient-Centered Oncology Care on Healthcare Utilization and Cost

Results of Search

We initially identified 3158 citations based on our search criteria and obtained 25 citations from other sources. As described in Fig. 7.2 (PRISMA form), there were 2038 remaining titles after removing duplicates. We reviewed the titles and abstracts for inclusion and 1704 were excluded as not meeting the criteria. Those excluded before obtaining full text papers were studies that were not original research studies, unrelated to patient-centered care, and were not applied to the treatment for cancer patients. We reviewed full text of 334 articles as broadly relevant. Of these, 324 were excluded, leaving a total of 10 articles. Those assessed in full text and excluded were ineligible in study designs, or were about a single patient-centered care intervention rather than the PCMH model as described above.

Study Characteristics

The final included articles consisted six cohort studies (Colligan et al., 2017a, 2017b; Goyal et al., 2014; Kohler et al., 2015; Sullivan et al., 2018; Wheeler et al., 2013) and four case series and case reports (Harper et al., 2015; Kuntz et al., 2014; Sprandio, 2010; Waters et al., 2015). Table 7.1 summarized the characteristics of the included studies. Patients were identified in the studies using International Classification of Disease, ninth edition (ICD-9) codes indicating active cancers. Among the ten included articles, the types of cancer included breast, lung, colorectal, lymphoma, pancreatic, thyroid, melanoma, male or female genitourinary cancers, or head or neck cancers in the analytic sample. Included studies mainly compared outcomes between cancer patients who received PCOC and usual type of care. Data sources included cancer registry data, claims data, chart and other administrative data, as well as self-report/survey data. Patients included patient who received care at physician office, hospitals, specialist, or oncology practice.

Study Quality Appraisal

We used the Downs and Black's Quality Index (Downs & Black, 1998) to assess the quality of each study. Based on the quality of reporting, internal validity (bias and confounding), study power, as well as external validity, an overall score and a level of quality appraisal was given to each study. As shown in Table 7.1, we scored three studies as high quality (scored above 23), and seven studies as medium quality (scored range from 12 to 22). Of those six cohort studies, three were scored as medium quality. All four studies for narrative summaries were graded as medium quality. In terms of major factors led to medium quality, internal bias and selection bias, such as lack of attempt made to blind study subjects, and incomprehensive adjustment for confounding in the analyses, were concluded in most studies with medium quality appraisal.

Attributes of Patient-Centered Oncology Care

Most studies appeared to implement the majority of six PCMH core attributes. Moreover, these included oncology care models addresses the extra steps involved in using a patient-centered approach to treat patients with cancer. We found that besides the core component of PCMH, three additional components related to oncology care were commonly implemented by most included studies, which were (1) telephone triage pathways to help first responders identify patient symptoms and ensure patients receive appropriate care (trained nurses utilized customized symptom management algorithms to ensure health problems were addressed appropriately and proactively managed to prevent unnecessary health service utilization) (Colligan et al., 2017a, 2017b; Harper et al., 2015; Kuntz et al., 2014; Sprandio, 2010; Sullivan et al., 2018; Waters et al., 2015); (2) standardized and evidence-based symptom management (Colligan et al., 2017a, 2017b; Goyal et al., 2014; Kohler et al., 2015; Kuntz et al., 2014; Sprandio, 2010); and (3) support patient navigation (Colligan et al., 2017b; Goyal et al., 2014; Kohler et al., 2015; Sprandio, 2010; Sullivan et al., 2018; Wheeler et al., 2013), such as coordinating referrals and assisting with transitions across settings and providers.

Adverse Healthcare Utilization

Six out of ten studies reported the outcomes of ED use (Colligan et al., 2017a, 2017b; Goyal et al., 2014; Kohler et al., 2015; Kuntz et al., 2014; Sprandio, 2010). Negative effect sizes denoted improvement when it came to ER utilization. Negative effects are found in three of four analytical studies (Colligan et al., 2017a, 2017b; Goyal et al., 2014), and only one study showed positive effect (Kohler et al., 2015) but with non-statistical significance. The meta-analyses were performed with a random effects model for assessing heterogeneity. The results of I^2 represented moderate heterogeneity (I^2 ranging 30–50% may represent moderate heterogeneity), however, the P value indicated that the evidence of heterogeneity of intervention effects was not statistically significant ($I^2 = 41.24\%$, $P = 0.17$). Overall effect size of four analytical studies was small and not statistically significant (standardized means difference

[SMD] = −0.023, $P = 0.103$). The highest effect was in Goyal et al. (2014, SMD = −0.083, $P = 0.001$). Publication bias was assessed by funnel plots and Egger's tests. The results showed that there was no statistical evidence of publication bias in the meta-analysis ($P = 0.491$). Among the two studies for narrative summaries, Kuntz et al. (2014) found the ER visits were lower among the patients who enrolled in the oncology medical home. Similarly, in Sprandio's study (2010), the ER referrals had decreased progressively since patients participated the oncology PCMH (Figs. 7.3 and 7.4).

Six studies assessed the inpatient use (Colligan et al., 2017a, 2017b; Goyal et al., 2014; Kohler et al., 2015; Kuntz et al., 2014; Sprandio, 2010). Negative effect sizes denoted improvement when it came to inpatient utilization. The negative effects were found in three (Colligan et al., 2017a; Goyal et al., 2014; Kohler et al., 2015) of four analytical studies (Colligan et al., 2017a, 2017b; Goyal et al., 2014; Kohler et al.,

Study name	Sample size	SMD (95%CI)	Weight(%)
Colligan (2017) a	3323	-0.083 (-0.131, 0.035)	41.05
Colligan (2017) b	1224	-0.011 (-0.090, 0.068)	30.67
Goyal (2014)	570	-0.048 (-0.213, 0.117)	12.70
Kohler(2015)	758	0.012 (-0.025, 0.050)	15.58
Overall		-0.023 (-0.050, 0.005)	100

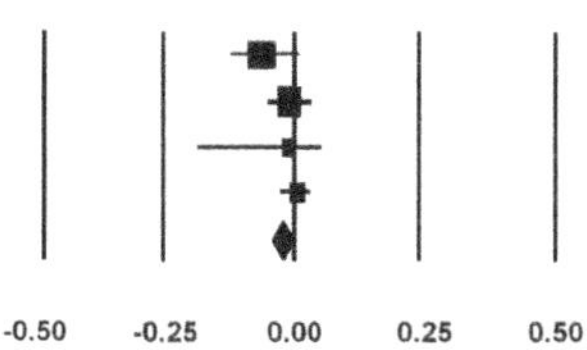

Fig. 7.3 Forest plot of effect sizes of ED visit. *Note* 1. A random-effects meta-analysis was used to incorporate heterogeneity among studies. 2. The direction of effect: the negative results indicate that an intervention works in reducing ER visits. 3. Colligan et al. (2017a, 2017b) were associated with the community oncology medical home (COME HOME) model; Goyal et al. (2014) and Kohler et al. (2015) were associated with the PCMH program of Community Care of North Carolina (CCNC)

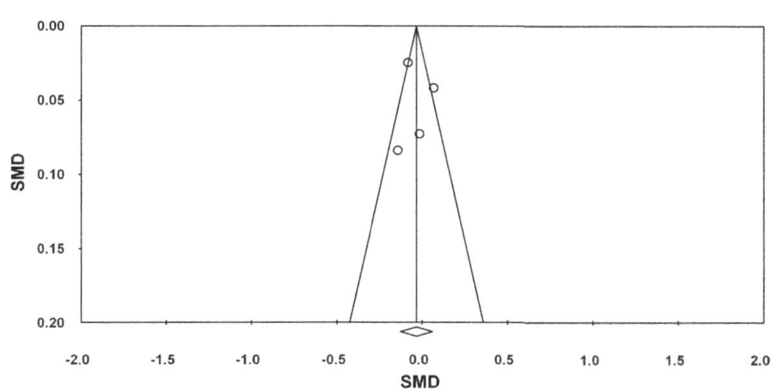

Fig. 7.4 Funnel plot of effect sizes of ED visits. *Note* Results of the Egger's test: $t = 0.288$, $p = 0.80$

2015). The only one study with positive effects (Colligan et al., 2017b) was not statistically significant. The overall effect size of four analytical studies was statistical significant (SMD = −0.027, $P = 0.049$). The results of I^2 represented substantial heterogeneity (I^2 ranging 50–90% may represent substantial heterogeneity), however, the P value indicated that the evidence of heterogeneity of intervention effects was not statistically significant ($I^2 = 72.57\%$, $P = 0.228$). Publication bias was assessed by funnel plots and Egger's tests, and there was no statistical evidence of publication bias in the meta-analysis ($P = 0.80$). Of the two studies for narrative summaries, Kuntz et al. (2014) found the numbers of the inpatient admissions were lower for patients who enrolled in the Michigan Oncology Medical Home Demonstration Project (MOMHDP), and Sprandio (2010) found a 16% reduction in overall hospital admissions since patients participated the oncology PCMH. Moreover, two studies reported outpatient use (Goyal et al., 2014; Kohler et al., 2015). Goyal et al. (2014) found nonsignificant association between PCMH enrollment and the outpatient visits. On the contrary, Kohler et al. (2015) found PCMH enrollment was associated with 0.53 more outpatient visits monthly (Figs. 7.5 and 7.6).

Cost

Four studies reported the costs (Colligan et al., 2017a, 2017b; Kohler et al., 2015; Kuntz et al., 2014). In general, patients who were involved in PCMH model cost less compared to their comparative, historic or other groups. Colligan et al. (2017a) found that the cost of the oncology medical home model was associated with a lower Medicare cost of $675 per patient per quarter through up to 3 years after the enrollment of the model ($P < 0.01$). In Colligan et al. (2017b), the oncology medical home was associated with a decreased total Medicare cost of $3346 in the last 90 days of life. In Kuntz et al. (2014), the oncology medical home reduced an average estimated cost savings of $550 per patient at the practices that participated in the first year of the demonstration project. However, there is one exception, showing a higher

Study name	Sample size	SMD (95%CI)	Weight(%)
Colligan (2017) a	3323	-0.084 (-0.132, -0.036)	41.05
Colligan (2017) b	1224	0.057 (-0.022, 0.136)	30.67
Goyal (2014)	570	-0.140 (-0.305, 0.025)	12.70
Kohler(2015)	758	-0.006 (-0.043, 0.031)	15.58
Overall		-0.027 (-0.055,-0.001)	100

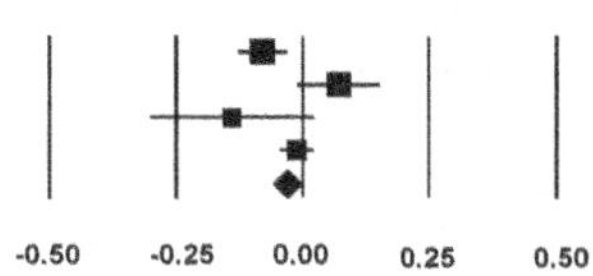

Fig. 7.5 Forest plot of effect sizes of hospitalizations. *Note* 1. A random-effects meta-analysis was used to incorporate heterogeneity among studies. 2. The direction of effect: the negative results indicate that an intervention works in reducing hospitalizations. 3. Colligan et al. (2017a, 2017b) were associated with the community oncology medical home (COME HOME) model; Goyal et al. (2014) and Kohler et al. (2015) were associated with the PCMH program of Community Care of North Carolina (CCNC)

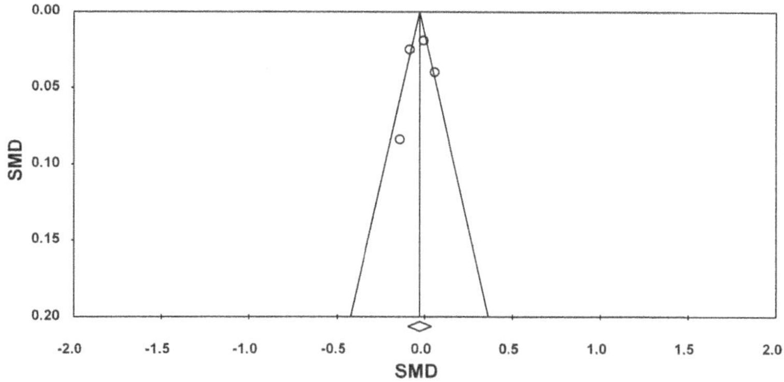

Fig. 7.6 Funnel plot of effect sizes of hospitalizations. *Note* Results of the Egger's test: $t = 0.835$, $p = 0.491$

cost. Kohler et al. (2015) found that in the first 15 months after diagnosis, enrollment in a PCMH was related to an increase of $429 in monthly average Medicaid spending.

Quality of Care and Patient Satisfaction

One included study reported the results of access of care (Wheeler et al., 2013), one included study reported the quality of end-of-life care (Sullivan et al., 2018) and two studies reported the patient satisfaction (Harper et al., 2015; Waters et al., 2015). In Wheeler et al. (2013), PCMH enrollment was significantly and positively related to the access of mammography ($P = 0.021$). Waters et al. (2015) found that patients were highly satisfied with the care they received in the PCMH project. Harper et al. (2015) found that patient satisfied with care in oncology medical home and felt comfortable with their plan of care.

7.5 The Impact of Patient-Centered Oncology Care on Healthcare Utilization and Cost

We reviewed studies evaluating PCMH models applied to oncology care in order to better understand the essential component of PCOC, whether their adoptions were associated with lower rates of ER visits and hospitalization, whether they were related to reduced health care costs, and whether they were helpful in improving patient experience. We found that PCOC patients had lower utilization of inpatient care. Overall positive effect of PCOC on ER use was small and not significant. In terms of cost and quality of care, our narrative summaries showed an overall positive direction, though we found limitations in individual study quality that precluded a meta-analysis.

Compared with previous reviews, our findings may draw different conclusions related to the utilization measures. For example, a systematic review in 2013 on

PCMH showed no effect on inpatient utilization among older adults with chronic conditions based on the results from five trials (Jackson et al., 2013). However, a recent systematic review and meta-analysis showed PCMH patients had lower utilization of emergency rooms (van den Berk-Clark et al., 2017) among low-income population. This may have implied that the patient-centered care model may have different effects among different populations with varying diseases (Kohler et al., 2015).

Our study also demonstrated that many of the core components of PCOC were being implemented across studies. Serving as decision support tools, the triage pathways help trained responders, such as nurses or physician assistants, to ask questions and use symptom management algorithms to determine if a cancer patient is having an emergency, if the patient should be seen for a same-day appointment, or should be given phone advice and scheduled for a follow-up visit (Colligan et al., 2017a, 2017b; Sprandio, 2010). For example, an included study by Sprandio (2010) found that more than 75% of all calls from triage system resulted in managing symptoms at home. About 10% resulted in a same-day visit and less than 5% resulted in an ER visit. Another component applied among most included studies were standardization of diagnosis and treatment pathways in compliance with evidence-based guidelines. Many current studies showed that clinical process standardization is not only a driver of value, but also a major driver of higher efficiency, better quality of care and health outcomes (Kuntz et al., 2014; Page et al., 2015; Waters et al., 2015). The last component of patient navigation generally has a broad scope; navigation services were provided in and between multiple settings, including hospitals, ERs, and patient's home. This component showed promise in reducing adverse health care utilization among cancer patients (Colligan et al., 2017a).

Also of interest are mixed outcomes which were observed when it came to utilization and cost-saving. Specifically, there was a small improvement in ER use. Compared with patients who received usual care, patients who received PCOC were more likely to get enhanced access to the clinic or navigator by the use of the triage system, and could take advantage of extended and weekend hours, which helped them get timely care and avoid unnecessary ER visits (Colligan et al., 2017a). There was improvement when it came to inpatient visits. Our study reported statistically significant findings in decreased inpatient admissions among patient-centered oncology patient group. Many avoidable inpatient admissions are rooted in difficulties that patients have accessing timely care in the primary care setting. Our findings suggested an important potential value of patient-centered care's efforts to improve coordination of cancer care (Goyal et al., 2014).

In terms of cost, our narrative summaries showed an overall positive direction in cost-savings. Among four studies reporting on health care spending, two cohort studies and one case series demonstrated reduced cost among PCOC groups, compared to the control groups. The key to controlling health care cost is the reduction and avoidance of unnecessary utilization and costs. Components of PCOC, such as patient triage and standard clinical pathways, can play an important role in shepherding patients through decision making and evidence-based symptom management to prevent unplanned hospitalizations and unneeded ER visits (Colligan et al., 2017a,

2017b; Kuntz et al., 2014). Additionally, under the PCOC, successful management of the financial risks, and maximizing global patient management based on appropriate accredited benchmarks can make oncology practices remain viable going forward (ASCO, 2014; McAneny, 2013).

Included studies had some substantial limitations. First of all, because PCOC models are composed of a "basket" of multiple features, and definitions for components were different among models, examining and standardizing model components is beyond the scope of this work. Second, the included studies using a cohort design did not achieve random assignment, which hindered the possibility to conclude causal inferences. However, utilizing randomization design in social and health service studies may bring out ethical issues. Future studies may choose an alternative strategy for overcoming this, such as one included study using propensity score matching, to control variables that could confound the exposure (Colligan et al., 2017a). Third, most included studies were based on the claims data and matched to cancer registry, which could cause a lack of reliable measures for controlling for cancer severity and stage. Fourth, due to PCOC at an early stage and limited number of literature on PCOC available, we did not set specific criteria for stages of cancer and types of settings. Future study may focus on the impact of PCOC on a specific stage of cancer care or within one type of setting where the interventions were implemented. Last, other factors may be associated with outcomes. Stratification involving the division of participants into subgroups with respect to categorical prognostic factors may use for a pooled estimate calculated across strata. However, the poor resolution in the measurement of confounders, e.g. co-morbidity assessed on a simple ordinal scale, precluded the possibility of conducting stratified analyses.

7.6 Practice Implications

To our knowledge, this is the first systematic review and meta-analysis on patient-centered oncology care (PCOC). The findings of this systematic review offer further evidence for meaningful practice, and have many policy and research implications. In fact, the results from our study shed light on PCOC's ability to support best-practice of cancer care. However, it is unclear whether the benefits gained from PCOC suggested by this review would offset challenges incurred by changes due to adoption of new models. For example, decreased hospitalization and increased outpatient use seems critical for strategic use of human and physical resources. Moreover, decreasing cost may translate to a reduced revenue to the health system. Moreover, allocating support and resources that are expected to help practitioners and administrators anticipate and respond to these changes due to the care model transition.

With regard to practice and policy implications, the lessons learned from the current synthesized evidence can further inform the implementation of these models. Many areas we identified as opportunities for improvement. From an administrator's perspective, although currently different types of PCOP models had many structures and processes in common, the PCOC practice standards varied widely across the practices. It is important to think broadly about how we can better use the main components of PCOC, and how we can make PCOP more standardized and documented. Some of the oncology-specific components were not established in a way that could produce documentation on demand. Besides, there were other areas, such as resources, infrastructure, leadership, cost versus benefit that need to be considered for implementing PCOC. These areas are facilitators for practice transformation. For example, infrastructure for health information exchange and care coordination across practices was needed to improve professional interactions and patient care transitions. Moreover, the PCOC model should be scaled up in more health care institutions that should be chosen to represent the diversity of the cancer treatment facilities (i.e., community hospitals, teaching hospitals, comprehensive cancer centers).

It is important to also recognize the advancement of currently implemented patient-centered oncology models. The patient-centered models started being applied to oncology care and its further use has been encouraged by the recent launch of multiple care models across the nation. For examples, MOMHDP (Kuntz et al., 2014) and Community Oncology Medical Home (COME HOME) (Colligan et al., 2017a, 2017b), have been widely adopted statewide or even nationwide, which implied these models' capacities of scaling up and sustainability. Our findings are very relevant to the CMS Oncology Care Model, which provides episode-based payments to practices for Medicare beneficiaries undergoing therapy, with quality performance accountability (CMS, 2016b). Under this model, participating practices are required to redesign themselves to include several aspects of PCOC (CMS, 2016a). Similar to PCOC, practices in the Oncology Care Model will provide therapies consistent with nationally recognized guidelines, and ensure timely access to appropriate care providers with real-time access to medical records (Clough & Kamal, 2015; CMS, 2016b). Moreover, these practices will use patient navigation to assist with transitions between health care settings and coordinating referrals (CMS, 2016b). PCOC offer valuable lessons on how to help patients avoid unnecessary utilization and thus reducing costs. The practices in the Oncology Care Model could benefit from adapting the PCOC's approach to design and implement core services to their context. On the other side, the Oncology Care Model provides an opportunity to test elements of the PCOC interventions on a larger scale, and with reformed payment mechanisms that could potentially support their increased implementation (Colligan et al., 2017b; Kline et al., 2015).

However, the currently available evidence is limited and in an earlier stage, more studies and evaluations are needed to determine the impact of the models on health care utilization, patients' health outcomes as well as cost. It is also crucial for collaborating to develop a core set of PCOC standards to enhance the focus, minimize the confusion, and shorten the timeline for adoption of new models. These unifications will enhance adoptability, and therefore the scalability of current models.

This chapter demonstrates that PCOC can be helpful with cancer patients, but the small number of relevant selected articles and the heterogeneity of those studies show that more rigorous research is expected to further investigate the model's effects on cancer patient care. It is important to use real-world evidence to support value in care delivery models. Providing high-quality care for cancer patients is challenging for several reasons, including the coordination of efforts from multiple providers, the use of several procedures and medications, coupled with continued follow-up and surveillance over time. The importance of innovative interventions and care models that can overcome these challenges, facilitate optimum care of cancer patients, and maintain quality of care given the increasing demand for care and shortages of providers. It has also been noted over time that, service, quality, and resource stewardship increases and will be further strengthened when considering the interrelationships among the three major entities in the service triad: the health care facilities, the providers, and the patient, as well as needs associated with health care performance. Reforms and policies should reflect these efforts, and the provision of such resources will promote the success of a sustainable transitions of cancer care. Given the emerging and promising evidence that PCOC is equipped to provide care management and coordination and improve communication, the authors of this review support that PCOC's role in addressing current challenges of delivering high-quality cancer care.

References

Ahmed, S., Shahid, R. K., & Gesy, K. (2015). Cancer care burden: Aiming at the Achilles heel. *Current Oncology, 22*(3), e134–e138. https://doi.org/10.3747/co.22.2252

American Cancer Society. (2013). *Economic impact of cancer*. Retrieved from www.cancer.org/cancer/cancerbasics/economic-impact-of-cancer

American Cancer Society. (2017). *Cancer facts & figures 2017*. American Cancer Society.

American Society of Clinical Oncology. (2014). Potential approaches to sustainable, long-lasting payment reform in oncology. *Journal of Oncology Practice, 10*(4), 254–258. https://doi.org/10.1200/JOP.2014.001267

Arend, J., Tsang-Quinn, J., Levine, C., & Thomas, D. (2012). The patient-centered medical home: History, components, and review of the evidence. *Mount Sinai Journal of Medicine, 79*(4), 433–450.

Centers for Medicare and Medicaid Services. (2016a). Oncology care model. Retrieved from https://innovation.cms.gov/initiatives/oncology-care/

Centers for Medicare and Medicaid Services. (2016b). Fact sheet: Oncology care model. Retrieved from https://www.cms.gov/Newsroom/MediaReleaseDatabase/Fact-sheets/2016-Fact-sheets-items/2016-06-29.html

Centers for Medicare and Medicaid Services. (2017). Key drivers and change package. Retrieved from https://innovation.cms.gov/Files/x/ocm-keydrivers-changepkg.pdf

Clough, J. D., & Kamal, A. H. (2015). Oncology care model: Short- and long-term considerations in the context of broader payment reform. *Journal of Oncology Practice, 11*(4), 319–321. https://doi.org/10.1200/JOP.2015.005777

Colligan, E. M., Ewald, E., Keating, N. L., Parashuram, S., Spafford, M., Ruiz, S., & Moiduddin, A. (2017a). Two innovative cancer care programs have potential to reduce utilization and spending. *Medical Care, 55*(10), 873–878. https://doi.org/10.1097/MLR.0000000000000795

Colligan, E. M., Ewald, E., Ruiz, S., Spafford, M., Cross-Barnet, C., & Parashuram, S. (2017b). Innovative oncology care models improve end-of-life quality, reduce utilization and spending. *Health Affairs (Millwood), 36*(3), 433–440. https://doi.org/10.1377/hlthaff.2016.1303

Collins, L. G., Wender, R., & Altshuler, M. (2010). An opportunity for coordinated cancer care: Intersection of health care reform, primary care providers, and cancer patients. *Cancer Journal, 16*(6), 606–613. https://doi.org/610.1097/PPO.1090b1013e318201fdac.

Downs, S. H., & Black, N. (1998). The feasibility of creating a checklist for the assessment of the methodological quality both of randomised and non-randomised studies of health care interventions. *Journal of Epidemiology and Community Health, 52*(6), 377–384.

Eagle, D., & Sprandio, J. (2012). A care model for the future: The oncology medical home. *Patient Education and Counseling, 87*(2), 206–211. https://doi.org/210.1016/j.pec.2011.1008.1010.

Edwards, B. K., Noone, A. M., Mariotto, A. B., Simard, E. P., Boscoe, F. P., Henley, S. J., Jemal, A., Cho, H., Anderson, R. N., Kohler, B. A., Eheman, C. R., & Ward, E. M. (2014). Annual report to the nation on the status of cancer, 1975–2010, featuring prevalence of comorbidity and impact on survival among persons with lung, colorectal, breast, or prostate cancer. *Cancer, 120*(9), 1290–1314. https://doi.org/10.1002/cncr.28509

Egger, M., Smith, G. D., Schneider, M., & Minder, C. (1997). Bias in meta-analysis detected by a simple, graphical test. *BMJ, 315*(7109), 629–634.

Goyal, R. K., Wheeler, S. B., Kohler, R. E., Lich, K. H., Lin, C. C., Reeder-Hayes, K., Meyer, A.-M., & Mayer, D. K. (2014). Health care utilization from chemotherapy-related adverse events among low-income breast cancer patients: Effect of enrollment in a medical home program. *North Carolina Medical Journal, 75*(4), 231–238.

Harper, J. L., De Costa, A. M., Garrett-Mayer, E., & Sterba, K. R. (2015). Incorporating patient satisfaction metrics in assessing multidisciplinary breast cancer care quality. *Southern Medical Journal, 108*(6), 372–376. https://doi.org/10.14423/SMJ.0000000000000300

Hewitt, M. E., Greenfield, S., Stovall, E., & Board, N. C. P. (2005). *From cancer patient to cancer survivor: Lost in transition*. National Academies Press.

Hoff, T., Weller, W., & DePuccio, M. (2012). The patient-centered medical home: A review of recent research. *Medical Care Research Review, 69*(6), 619–644. https://doi.org/10.1177/1077558712447688

Huang, X., & Rosenthal, M. B. (2014). Transforming specialty practice—The patient-centered medical neighborhood. *New England Journal Medicine, 370*(15), 1376–1379. https://doi.org/10.1056/NEJMp1315416

Jackson, G. L., Powers, B. J., Chatterjee, R., Bettger, J. P., Kemper, A. R., Hasselblad, V., Dolor, R. J., Irvine, R. J., Heidenfelder, B. L., Kendrick, A. S., Gray, R., & Williams, J. W. (2013). Improving patient care. The patient centered medical home. A systematic review. *Annals of Internal Medicine, 158*(3), 169–178. https://doi.org/10.7326/0003-4819-158-3-201302050-00579

Kline, R. M., Bazell, C., Smith, E., Schumacher, H., Rajkumar, R., & Conway, P. H. (2015). Centers for Medicare and Medicaid Services: Using an episode-based payment model to improve oncology care. *Journal of Oncology Practice, 11*(2), 114–116. https://doi.org/10.1200/JOP.2014.002337

Kohler, R. E., Goyal, R. K., Lich, K. H., Domino, M. E., & Wheeler, S. B. (2015). Association between medical home enrollment and health care utilization and costs among breast cancer patients in a state Medicaid program. *Cancer, 121*(22), 3975–3981. https://doi.org/10.1002/cncr.29596. Epub 2015 Aug 19.

Kuntz, G., Tozer, J. M., Snegosky, J., Fox, J., & Neumann, K. (2014). Michigan oncology medical home demonstration project: First-year results. *Journal of Oncology Practice, 10*(5), 294–297. https://doi.org/10.1200/JOP.2013.001365. Epub 2014 Jul 1.

Liang, H., Tao, L., Ford, E. W., Beydoun, M. A., & Eid, S. M. (2020). The patient-centered oncology care on health care utilization and cost: A systematic review and meta-analysis. *Health Care Manage Review, 45*(4), 364–376.

Liang, H., Zhu, J., Kong, X., Beydoun, M. A., Wenzel, J. A., & Shi, L. (2017). The patient-centered care and receipt of preventive services among older adults with chronic diseases: A nationwide cross-sectional study. *Inquiry, 54*, 46958017724003. https://doi.org/10.1177/0046958017724003

McAneny, B. L. (2013). The future of oncology? Come home, the oncology medical home. *American Journal of Managed Care, 19*(1 Spec No), cover, SP41-42.

McManus, L. S. (2017). *The patient-centered medical home and diabetes mellitus outcomes: A systematic review*. Retrieved from http://scholarworks.waldenu.edu/cgi/viewcontent.cgi?article=4413&context=dissertations

Moher, D., Liberati, A., Tetzlaff, J., Altman, D. G., & Group, P. (2009). Preferred reporting items for systematic reviews and meta-analyses: The PRISMA statement. *PLoS Medicine, 6*(7), e1000097. https://doi.org/10.1371/journal.pmed.1000097

National Cancer Institute. (2016). *Navigating cancer care*. Retrieved from https://www.cancer.net/navigating-cancer-care/older-adults/when-cancer-not-your-only-health-concern

National Cancer Institute. (2018). *Cancer statistics*. Retrieved from https://www.cancer.gov/about-cancer/understanding/statistics

National Committee for Quality Assurance. (2011). *NCQA patient-centered medical home 2011: Health care that revolves around you*. Retrieved from http://www.ncqa.org/Portals/0/Programs/Recognition/2011PCMHbrochure_web.pdf

National Committee for Quality Assurance. (2013). *Patient-centered specialty practice recognition*. Retrieved from https://www.ncqa.org/Portals/0/Newsroom/2013/PCSP%20Launch/PCSPR%202013%20White%20Paper%203.26.13%20formatted.pdf

Page, R. D., Newcomer, L. N., Sprandio, J. D., & McAneny, B. L. (2015). The patient-centered medical home in oncology: From concept to reality. *American Society of Clinical Oncology Educational Book*, e82–e89.

Patient-Centered Primary Care Collaborative (PCPCC). (2012). Pilots and demonstrations, joint principles of the patient-centered medical home. Retrieved from http://www.pcpcc.net/content/joint-principles-patient-centered-medical-home

Reibling, N. (2016). The patient-centered medical home: How is it related to quality and equity among the general adult population? *Medical Care Research Review, 73*(5), 606–623. https://doi.org/10.1177/1077558715622913

Rosenthal, T. C. (2008). The medical home: Growing evidence to support a new approach to primary care. *Journal of American Board of Family Medicine, 21*(5), 427–440.

Shi, L., Lee, D. C., Chung, M., Liang, H., Lock, D., & Sripipatana, A. (2017). Patient-centered medical home recognition and clinical performance in US community health centers. *Health Services Research, 52*(3), 984–1004.

Sprandio, J. D. (2010). Oncology patient-centered medical home and accountable cancer care. *Community Oncology, 7*(12), 565–572.

StataCorp. (2011). *Stata statistical software: Release 12*. StataCorp LP.

Sullivan, D. R., Ganzini, L., Lapidus, J. A., Hansen, L., Carney, P. A., Osborne, M. L., Fromme, E. K., Izumi, S., & Slatore, C. G. (2018). Improvements in hospice utilization among patients with advanced-stage lung cancer in an integrated health care system. *Cancer, 124*(2), 426–433.

van den Berk-Clark, C., Doucette, E., Rottnek, F., Manard, W., Prada, M. A., Hughes, R., Lawrence, T., & Schneider, F. D. (2017). Do patient-centered medical homes improve health behaviors, outcomes, and experiences of low-income patients? A systematic review and meta-analysis. *Health Services Research*. https://doi.org/10.1111/1475-6773.12737

Waters, T. M., Webster, J. A., Stevens, L. A., Li, T., Kaplan, C. M., Graetz, I., & McAneny, B. L. (2015). Community oncology medical homes: Physician-driven change to improve patient care and reduce costs. *Journal of Oncology Practice, 11*(6), 462–467. https://doi.org/10.1200/JOP.2015.005256. Epub 2015 Jul 28.

Wender, R. C., & Altshuler, M. (2009). Can the medical home reduce cancer morbidity and mortality. *Primary Care, 36*(4), 845–858.

Wheeler, S. B., Kohler, R. E., Goyal, R. K., Lich, K. H., Lin, C. C., Moore, A., Smith, T. W., Melvin, C. L., Reeder-Hayes, K., & Domino, M. E. (2013). Is medical home enrollment associated with receipt of guideline-concordant follow-up care among low-income breast cancer survivors? *Annals of Oncology, 24*(9), 2324–2329. https://doi.org/10.1093/annonc/mdt2195. Epub 2013 May 23.

Wilper, A. P., Woolhandler, S., Lasser, K. E., McCormick, D., Bor, D. H., & Himmelstein, D. U. (2008). A national study of chronic disease prevalence and access to care in uninsured U.S. adults. *Annals of Internal Medicine, 149*(3), 170–176.

Chapter 8
Policy Implications and Discussions

8.1 Introduction

The goal of the book was to improve understandings of the relationship between the receipt of patient-centered care and disparities in accessing selected preventive services, cancer care as well as the health outcomes in the United States. The study had two aims, which were to: (1) assess the associations between the receipt of PCC and chronic management among older adults, including receipt of preventive screening and health education for chronic diseases, as well as oncology care; (2) assess the associations between the receipt of PCC and chronic disease health outcomes among older adults, including patient perceived health status and incidence of adverse utilization events. The study's conceptual model integrated Donabedian's structure, process, and outcome model to construct the study design, and applied the Aday and Andersen's framework to select covariates that are related to the experience of PCC. A secondary analysis was conducted using the full-year consolidated Medical Expenditure Panel Survey Household Component Data Files Year 2009 through 2013.

This chapter demonstrates the key findings relative to the existing literature and discusses the policy as well as public health implications. First, we summarize the key findings for the study and for each specific aim, and then discuss how these findings relate to the existing literature and what policy implications can be derived. Next, we provide an overall discussion across all the study aims and explain the understanding how the overall study can inform the public health field. Then we address the limitations of the study, and end the chapter with suggestions for future research and a conclusion with respect to the whole study.

H. Liang, *The Impact of Patient-Centered Care*,
https://doi.org/10.1007/978-981-16-3968-5_8

8.2 Summary of the Key Findings

Analyses from this chapter revealed the impact of PCC on elderly chronic disease patients' health experiences, process of care, and health outcomes. PCC measures captured similar trends for most of the ten health process measures and four health outcome measures, that is, the PCC group having the best healthcare performance as well as health outcomes. This chapter presents the implications from results for the two aims of the study, which inform whether the receipt of PCC will increase preventive screening and health education for older adults with chronic conditions, and whether the receipt of PCC will be associated with greater patient perceived health status and fewer adverse healthcare utilization events.

The results from bivariate and multivariate analyses confirmed the Hypothesis 1.1 and 1.2. Across the all ten measures of preventive care, the unadjusted analysis revealed sizable disparities in receiving eight types of preventive screening and two types of health education among three different PCC groups. PCC and partial PCC patients were significantly more likely to receive each of the eight preventive screenings as well as the two types of health education. The result of each comparison was significant at $P < 0.05$. Similar to the findings from the bivariate analyses, even after control for individual and institutional characteristics, PCC and partial PCC groups were still found to be more likely than the non-PCC group to receiving preventive care screening and health education.

The hypothesis 2.1 was also confirmed by our analyses. Unadjusted proportions and adjusted analysis indicated differences existed for both physical and mental health status depending on whether the respondent having PCC, having partial PCC or not having PCC. However, the results regarding hospitalization and ER visits did not support my hypothesis 2.2. According to the results from the unadjusted analyses, the significant differences of hospitalization and ER visits were not observed across three types of PCC groups. The adjusted results also showed PCC status did not significantly affect the hospitalization and ER visits after individual predisposing, enabling, and need as well as system covariates are controlled for.

Across three attributes of PCC, those are the whole person care, the patient engagement and the enhanced access, the multivariate analyses showed varied results. Specifically, the whole person care attribute increased the odds of receiving seven types of preventive screenings. The patient engagement attribute increased the odds of receiving six types of preventive screening, the healthy diet education and the odds of perceiving good mental health status. The enhanced access attribute increased the odds of receiving two types of health screening, the odds of perceiving good physical health status, and the odds of having fewer ER visits.

8.3 Discussions of Findings and Policy Implications

In this section, we summary the key findings for each specific aim, and then discuss how these findings relate to the existing literature and what policy implications can be derived.

8.3.1 Discussion for the Aim 1: Patient-Centered Care and Preventive Care Services

The results from the analyses for Aim 1 indicates that the receipt of preventive care services varies significantly according to PCC status. In general, respondents from PCC and partial PCC groups are able to receive better preventive care services than the non-PCC respondents. Although respondents having higher socioeconomic status (SES) are more likely to receive more comprehensive care, this study has controlled for these factors and still demonstrates that the receipt of preventive screening and health education for chronic conditions varies according to whether the respondents were having PCC.

This finding suggests the basis of PCC is distinct from the traditional practice, and it not only achieve the main features of primary care—first contact, continuity, comprehensiveness and coordination—but also better fulfill patient needs and respect for patients' values. In contrast to the disease-focused and physician-centered care that centers on the health provider as the sole source of control and treat a disease without attention to the values of the patients, PCC tend to identify, respect, and care about patients' differences, expressed needs, values, and preferences, and to provide care that reflects the whole person. Therefore, these core focus of PCC provides the foundation for the long-term management of chronic conditions, which may have impact on the timely implementing strategies to identify, control and reduce risk factors for patients and to improve patients' access to appropriate preventive care services.

From a public policy perspective, it is important not only to promote the PCC model in a variety of healthcare settings, but also important to incorporate the PCC into specific vulnerable subgroups of population, such as the chronically ill older adults. This policy implication has direct relevance to the current Health Home program. The Section 2703 of the ACA created an optional Medicaid State Plan benefit for states to provide Health Homes for enrollees with multiple chronic conditions. The CMS expected states health home providers to integrate all primary, acute, behavioral health, and long-term services to treat chronic disease patients under a "whole-person" philosophy.

The differences in the receipt of preventive care services between partial PCC and non-PCC groups are mostly consistent with those observed between PCC and non-PCC groups. However, comparisons of the receipt of preventive care services of respondents from PCC and partial PCC yield that higher level of PCC is associated with superior preventive care, suggesting that more components of PCC in combination may yield improvements in preventive care, and practices will best sustain the PCC model when they adopt the most comprehensive components of PCC.

The study also indicates that the association between each of PCC attributes and the receipt of preventive care services. The most significant contribution that PCC attributes made in preventive screening is the whole person care attribute, which is associated with higher odds in getting seven out of eight types of preventive screenings. Although the magnitudes of the differences for some of these measures were small, the seven out of eight measures were broad enough and our findings provided a comprehensive representation throughout the nation, which provided sufficient power to detect the difference and imply the clinical significance. It is possible that the whole-person care approach could apply disease prevention and behavioral change principles appropriate by coordinating care in a patient-centered manner, and therefore make great strides to solve a broad range of health problems and toward achieving improved access to preventive services for specific populations (Bechtel & Ness, 2010; Ferrante et al., 2010). Our findings were consistent with a previous study that identified barriers of colorectal cancer screening among safety-net primary care clinics, in which the "whole-person approach" to the patients were showed as one of the promoters of colorectal cancer screening (O'Malley et al., 2004).

In terms of health education measures, patient engagement is the only attribute of PCC significantly associated with higher odds in getting the healthy diet educations, presumably because the patient's greater engagement in healthcare contributes to significant improvements in communication between patients and healthcare providers. Healthcare providers adopt PCC by clearly informing, listening to and communicating with patients and continuously advocate wellness, healthy lifestyles and disease prevention, which all furtherly improve the patients' access to health education as well as other preventive care services (Carman et al., 2013; Coulter, 2012; Michie et al., 2009; Roter et al., 2001).

In the comparison of the impact on the receipt of preventive care services between PCC status and each of the PCC attributes, we found that the adoption of various interdependent-PCC attributes as a whole rather than in increments were associated with more remarkable performance in preventive care. This finding suggests the multiple components of PCC are highly interdependent. Each component, when implemented, may affect throughout the medical process, and involving all the individual roles. The whole person care attribute is the most important aspects of the PCC, and evidence of the success of such approaches has been instrumental in guiding efforts to incorporate the other two attributes into PCC delivery. PCC Interventions that combined whole-person care attribute with other attributes were significantly more effective than the PCC interventions with separate attributes. The combinatory efforts can be associated with better chronic diseases management. It is important for healthcare providers who best sustained PCC model to implement as more components of PCC as possible, that are, to designate a personal physician for each patient, to provide accessible, comprehensive and continuous first contact, to coordinate with the care offered by other providers, and to engage patients in shared decision making. From a patient perspective, this means to contract a regular provider whose role is in total care for patients and who knows patients well. Patients can get timely access to well-coordinated care, to closely engage in their care and share their own thoughts with healthcare providers in medical decision making. From a practice perspective, adopting PCC require whole-practice redesign and transformation, which is much more than a series of incremental changes (Kilo et al., 2010), and demands a costly investment. Further studies by using experiment or quasi-experiment design are needed to demonstrate causality between PCC interventions and outcomes, and by using cost-effectiveness analysis to justify the PCC interventions' cost-effectiveness. Transformation includes improved appointment scheduling system, "after-hour" access arrangements, an off-hours telephone service, effective coordination across several healthcare providers, initiating team-based care, implementing point of care, quality improvement activities, innovations in practice management, creative strategies for patient engagement and shared decision making, as well as multiple uses of health information systems.

To our knowledge, this study is one of the first examining the association of PCC status in its entirety and in its individual attributes with a broad range of preventive services, and specifically focus on the older adults with chronic conditions. Previous studies, however, have demonstrated the association between the receipt of preventive care services and PCC status or attributes, neither the target population defined as older adults with chronic conditions nor the nationally representative estimates is well investigated. Using a random sample of facility-level Veterans Satisfaction Survey, Flach et al. assessed the relationship between PCC attributes and the provision of preventive services, and found that the two attributes of PCC, defined as improved communication and continuity of care, were associated with increased provision of preventive services, while other attributes were not significantly associated to receipt of preventive services (Flach et al., 2004). On the basis of a cross-sectional patient and practice member surveys conducted in 24 primary care offices in New Jersey, Ferrante et al. found that higher global PCMH scores were associated with receipt of preventive services, mainly resulting from positive associations with the whole-person care and personal physician attributes (Ferrante et al., 2010), which was consistent with our findings that the whole-person attribute of PCC was associated with higher odds of getting seven types of preventive services. Several studies demonstrate the relevance of PCC in other healthcare settings and investigate the association between the form of PCC and other process measurements. For example, a randomized controlled trial of 866 adult type 2 diabetes patients demonstrated a patient-centered diabetes care intervention increased the patient's self-management of the disease (Williams et al., 2007). Another eight-month patient-centred intervention aimed at identifying people with mild mental health problems showed the impact of PCC on helping patient to identify lifestyle mental health at early stage and improve the rate of patient requesting for help (Calveley et al., 2009). The other evidence highlight the impact of PCC on other process measures, including HIV patients' adherence to medication treatment regimens (Roberts, 2002), the follow-up treatment for cancer (Kahn et al., 2007; Zolnierek & Dimatteo, 2009), and the receipt of palliative care (Yedidia, 2007). Although these studies were not directly comparable with our work, the associations between PCC models/attributes and the provision of preventive services were overall points in a same positive direction, which were consistent with our findings.

8.3.2 Discussion for the Aim 2: Patient-Centered Care and Health Outcome Measures

The results from the analyses for the Aim 2 indicate that the perceived physical and mental health status varies significantly according to PCC status. However, there were no statistically significant associations between PCC status and adverse healthcare utilization events, measured by the hospitalization and ER visits. In general, respondents from PCC and partial PCC groups are more likely to perceive excellent/very good/good physical health status and mental health status than the non-PCC respondents. Although the higher SES may contribute to better perceived health status, our study has controlled for these factors and still demonstrates that the respondents' perceived health status varies according to whether the respondents were having PCC.

The findings suggests that the approaches/attributes of PCC are emerging to improve chronic disease patient's healthcare experience by timely responding and addressing their evolving physical and mental health needs. Specifically, the whole person care approach enabling patients to contract a regular provider whose role is in total care (routine healthcare, preventive services, referrals, and care for ongoing health problems) for patients and who knows patients well, which may has impact on reducing the fragmentation of care and coping with the challenges of delivering chronic care to patients with complex needs (Stange, 2009). The patient engagement in care is important in building trust among patients and providers by promoting communication and shared decision making, which can be one of the effective ways to help patient generate commitment to treatment plans (Coulter & Ellins, 2007). The enhanced access appears very helpful in eliminating barriers to care from the supply side and therefore encouraging patients to seek care during the early stage of their disease and furtherly to reduce risk and improve health (Jackson et al., 2013; Waxmonsky et al., 2011). Therefore, these PCC components may help the elderly chronic disease patient well manage their conditions and achieve both physical and mental health status.

The finding also suggests that self-reported measures from patients, such as perceived health and mental health status used in this study, are expected to play a more important role in evaluating performance of new healthcare models and interventions. The reason is that these measures are reported by the patients, which can appropriately provide evidence to support the specific model is effective in producing value for patients (Ahmed et al., 2012; Lohr & Zebrack, 2009; Valderas et al., 2008). This policy implication has direct relevance to the current plans developed by the Department of Health and Human Services' Office of the National Coordinator for

Health Information Technology (ONC) to incorporate self-reported measures into meaningful use standards (Chung & Basch, 2015; Wu et al., 2013).

Our hypothesis 2.2—the receipt of PCC will be associated with fewer adverse healthcare utilization events—was not confirmed by our analyses. One possible explanation is that PCC interventions were mostly too short to contribute to the hospital or ER avoidance. One other explanation might be that PCC model is generally targeted to improve primary care delivery, which means it still lacks effective strategies in this model to coordination with inpatient services, and to well manage post-discharge care and control the re-hospitalization. According to a study published in the New England Journal of Medicine, the author found that of the 12 million Medicare recipients in 2009, 19% of them were re-hospitalized within 30 days and 34% within 90 days (Jencks et al., 2009). The bigger issue with incomplete following care after discharge and re-hospitalizations might lead to higher rate of hospitalization and ER visits.

The study also indicates that the association between each of PCC attributes and the health outcome measures. Similar to the findings from the multivariate analyses on the association between PCC status and the health outcome measures, no PCC attributes were found to be associated with hospitalization. It is possible that some of the intervening factors may not be captured in MEPS, such as acuity and severity of illness, as well as differential application of PCC, etc. We cannot control the severity or acuity of the disease due to the limitation of the secondary data, but this might explain why the PCC is not associated with the better outcome variable. As the patients with severe conditions may have more medical visits and be more likely to receive PCC, that means the entries of PCC among patients with different severity of illness are different, and more severe patients are more likely to experience hospitalization. The other explanation might be the higher rate of re-hospitalizations. In terms of patient perceived health status, patient engagement attribute of PCC significantly associated with higher odds in patient perceiving good mental health status, presumably because the improved patient engagement may lead to close relationship between patients and healthcare providers, and so providers would be more likely to screen, identify and outreach people with mental health problems, and to motivate patients to play an active role in mental health self-management (Hibbard & Greene, 2013; Salyer et al., 2009). The results also show that enhanced access is significantly associated with higher odds in patient perceiving good physical health status. It is possible that enhanced access contributes to significant improvements in scheduling options and ensuring 24/7 continuous access to care, which all furtherly improve the patient experience of care as well as their perceived health status (Leibowitz et al., 2003; Murray & Berwick, 2003; O'Connell et al., 2001). In contrast to the finding from the multivariate analysis on the association between PCC status and the ER visits, one PCC attribute—the enhance access—were found to be associated with fewer ER visits. This finding suggests that the enhanced access may prevent some ER visits that occurred due to the lack of access to timely primary care. The enhance access component of PCC plays a fundamental role in reducing the health risk as well as avoidable ER visits by delivering first-contact, continuous and comprehensive primary care to the chronic disease patients with high demand of healthcare services at their early stage of diseases and conditions.

In the comparison of different impact on the health outcome measures between PCC status and PCC attributes, we found that the whole person care attribute of PCC is not individually associated with any of the four health outcome measures. This finding suggests that patients who have a regular provider for their total care did not necessarily contribute to better health outcomes. Only when the key PCC components achieve successful integration, the PCC may accomplish more notable improvement in health outcomes.

Our findings for the hypothesis 2.1 are consistent with other studies that compare the health outcomes between PCC and non-PCC patients. On the basis of a cross-sectional data from the cancer patients at a New England urban safety net hospital, Radwin et al. found that the implementation of patient-centered nursing intervention was associated with good general health, mainly resulting from positive associations with the intervention of individualized care and sense of well-being (Radwin et al., 2013). Another cross-sectional study of 200 army soldiers and their families showed a significant positive association between a better mental health status and access attribute of PCC (Moore et al., 2013).

The findings regarding the impact of PCC on hospitalization and ER visits are mixed. Our hypothesis 2.2 that the receipt of patient-centered care will be associated with fewer adverse healthcare utilization events is not confirmed by the analyses, however, it is consistent with the findings from some other studies. For example, by conducting a random controlled trail of 322 patients with advanced cancer in a rural cancer center in New Hampshire, Bakitas et al. found that nurse conducting PCC interventions regarding patient engagement and whole person care were not associated with the reduction of hospitalization and ER visits (Bakitas et al., 2009). The findings highlighted the complexity of chronic conditions management among older adults, and the possibility of mediate effect from other factors, such as the re-hospitalization due to the weak post-discharge care (Bakitas et al., 2009).

8.4 Overall Impact of the Findings

8.4.1 The Implications for Older Adults with Chronic Conditions

For decades, the US healthcare system has fallen short in its effort to adapt to the changing needs of the population and to provide them high-value healthcare services (Arend et al., 2012). In ongoing effort to reform the national health care system, PCC is recognized as a promising approach of care to better align care process with patient needs by combining traditional strength of primary care with innovative practice arrangements (Arend et al., 2012). Although PCC enjoys broad support by multiple stakeholders and a considerable number of studies on the effect of PCC are existed, there is no nationwide evidence to our knowledge that particularly focused on the benefits of PCC for the older adults with chronic conditions. Our study filled this specific knowledge gaps by investigating the impact of PCC on this vulnerable subpopulation and including a broad array of measures.

In addition, our study aims to cope with the demographic transition and the shifting burden of disease, which has several implications for public health. The world has experienced a demographic change in the distribution of population towards older ages. In the United States, the population aged 65 and over is projected to be 83.7 million in 2050, almost double its estimated population of 43.1 million in 2012 (Ortman et al., 2014). The age structure will experience a shift from 13.7% of the population aged 65 and over in 2012 to 20.3% in 2030 (U.S. Ortman et al., 2014). At the same time, the global burden of disease is shifting from infectious diseases to non-communicable diseases. Correspondingly, our study shed light on this shift away from focus on episodic acute care to focus on health management, and informed that long-term care management is central to the defined populations living with chronic conditions. Chronic conditions differ from acute conditions on a variety of important dimensions. Acute conditions usually have a short period of time of onset, while the chronic conditions generally require a lengthy duration of treatment, and the threat of conditions is long-lasting and ongoing, which may affect patient's life on a variety of the aspects, including physical, psychological social and economic dimensions. However, the current US healthcare system is operated primarily to react to acute conditions and ignore the complex health needs of chronic disease patients (Tinetti & Fried, 2004). The system principally responds to patient's chronic conditions only when the patient's symptoms occur. Therefore, the current system fails to provide timely care management to the chronic disease patients and overlooked patient's long-term health needs, the influence of lifestyle factors, comorbidity screening and prevention, and the vital role of mental health support. Our study revealed the promise of the PCC, which could target the elderly with chronic conditions, and optimally provide them PCC of long-term monitoring, full complement of services and continuous support.

Moreover, our study capture the current paradigm shift from the traditional provider-driven care model to patient actively engaged care model, and highlighted the patient's role in the chronic disease management, which is very critical for the chronically illed older patients. In traditional care model, healthcare providers were the center of the whole medical process, and may communicate inadequately with patients. Therefore they were more likely to have incomplete information about the patient's condition and treatment history, or providing care that the person may not want. Under the PCC model, patients are more likely to engage in their care and share their thoughts with providers about the treatment decisions. Therefore, healthcare providers will be easier to identify patient's needs, and will treat patient as a whole. From the patient's perspective, they will be the center during the whole process of PCC, and will be more effective in managing their chronic conditions. Such transitions of patient's role in the care would overcome the current fragmented and poorly coordinated chronic care, and furtherly improve chronically illed older patients' health outcomes.

8.4.2 Implications from the Comparison Between Our Findings with Literature

The evidence for the impact of PCC is in general points in a positive direction (Arend et al., 2012). The findings from this study answered the two research questions-whether the adoption of PCC has association with superior receipt of preventive services, and whether the adoption of PCC has association with improved health outcomes, which were critical for deriving insights for the PCC future development. The findings in our study supported positive associations between the PCC and the receipt of preventive care services as well as perceived health status, and showed no association between PCC and the hospitalization as well as ER visits.

Incorporating a broad range of preventive services measures into evaluation is considered a key indicator for rigorous assessment of PCC. The findings in our study supported positive associations between the PCC and the receipt of multiple types of preventive care services. The findings correspond to the previous studies (Ferrnante et al., 2010; Markovitz et al., 2015; Sarfaty et al., 2011). In the traditional provider-driven care model, more preventive screenings were provided when a patient was seeing a physician for a health problem. Under such situation, fewer opportunities and less time were available for the preventive services delivery. The model had the limitations in addressing full range of preventive health need of older adults with chronic conditions (Sarfaty et al., 2011). However, the PCC model overcome this drawback by actively engaging patient in their care and tailoring to the patient's needs, and therefore providing planned preventive services through a dedicated preventive health visits (Sarfaty et al., 2011). This explanation is also confirmed by our findings regarding the impact of PCC attributes: the attribute of whole person care has the most notable impact on increasing the receipt of receiving preventive screenings services. Patients receiving whole person care enable patients to contract a regular provider whose role is in total care, which contributes to more planned preventive health visits (Ferrnante et al., 2010; Sarfaty et al., 2011). Moreover, the patient engagement attribute also has the comparable impact on increasing the receipt of receiving preventive screenings services, but also contributes to receiving healthy diet education and perceiving good mental health status, which corresponds to the outcome previously reported: patient's perceptions of patient engagement did predict better emotional health (Stewart et al., 2000).

Our findings revealed no association between PCC and the hospitalization as well as ER visits. This finding was at least consistent with our expectation and contrary to other studies showing that PCC in primary care practice is associated with fewer hospitalization and ER visits (Nelson et al., 2014; Reid et al., 2009, 2010). Compared with Reid et al.'s studies, in which a quasi-experimental, two-group, before-and-after evaluation over two years was used to gauge the PCC's impact on utilization measures, our study did not have the opportunity to conduct pre-post testing and adjust for patient's disease severity, such as the diagnosis-based DxCG case-mix score used in Reid et al.'s studies. Such situation in our study may lead to some of the intervening factors cannot be captured in MEPS, like the severity of illness mentioned above. Patients with severe conditions may have more medical visits and be more likely to receive PCC, however, they may also be more likely to experience hospitalization or ER visit. This limitation in data may partially explain the unexpected results from our study. Moreover, a significant body of evidence indicates that process improvement lead to improved performance (Brownson et al., 1999; Hillestad et al., 2005; Morey et al., 2002). In our study, by using Donabedian framework, we clearly showed the relationships among the PCC-related structure, process and outcome variables. Therefore, if we could control all possible confounding variables, we would hypothesize that our positive association between process measures and PCC may extrapolate to positive results in health outcome measures.

8.4.3 The Generalizability of the Research Findings and Policy Implications

According to the WHO, public health refers to "all organized measures to prevent disease, promote health, and prolong life among the population as a whole. Its activities aim to provide conditions in which people can be healthy and focus on entire populations, not on individual patients or diseases". Like many other fields, public health has tended to rely on scientific knowledge to identify its problem, and require policy change to guide its development. The current research is subject to target the health needs of a specific vulnerable subpopulation, older adults with chronic conditions, and to evaluate the impact of PCC on improving health and well-being (Link, 1998). This study explicitly revealed that PCC have impact on well delivering care to the elderly with significant burden of chronic conditions in the United States. Findings from this study revealed implications for the future of health services research in the related field, and contributed to the existing evidence by proposing valid and replicable measures of PCC that could be assessed among older and chronically ill patient. The generalizability of the study was greatly enhanced by the national representativeness of the MEPS sample.

Transformation from current paradigm of practice into PCC necessitates tremendous investment. Although the overall impact of our findings are promising, policy makers may look beyond statistical significance for evidence of a clinically meaningful differences. Clinical significance is a subjective judgment and can't be determined by a single study. Therefore, our study along with other related evidence may play a viable role in promoting decision making to change the current practice. Building capacity for practice transformation may face formidable hurdles and require a wide range of efforts. At such, immediate initiatives might be needed to involve the coordinated care to meet patient's total healthcare needs, including routine or minor health problems, preventive healthcare, referrals to other health professionals and ongoing health problems (Cronholm et al., 2013). As for the patient engagement in care, it may requires healthcare providers' direct and in-the-moment efforts to promote interactions and communications with patients (Nutting et al., 2009; Wagner et al., 2012). With respect to the enhanced access, transformation is expected in information technology as well as the healthcare team partnership. The delivery of PCC can be well facilitated by registries, health information exchange and other means to assure that chronic disease patients get timely care when they need. Moreover, creating high-functioning health provider teams will help with overcoming the shortage of personnel (Cronholm et al., 2013). At the same time, using open scheduling, expanding hours and providing new options for communication between patients and their providers are also essential to achieve enhanced access for the elderly chronic disease patients (Crabtree et al., 2010; Nutting et al., 2009; Wagner et al., 2012).

8.5 Study Limitations

Our findings should be considered in light of certain limitations. First, our empirical sections adopts statistical models to capture the associations between the independent variables and dependent variables. However, the sequence of events cannot be determined. Therefore, it's difficult to make causal inferences from the analyses due the cross-sectional nature of the analyses.

Second, although multiple measures in our study showed statistically significant, the magnitude of the effect for several measures were not clinically meaningful, such as blood pressure check and perceived mental health status. Such lack of clinical significance may be due to the "ceiling effects", which means the overall percentage of measures were quite high and the effect of PCC interventions was underestimated, because the percentage can't differentiate between very high and somewhat high levels. Furthermore, even if the small differences were clinically meaningful, they would not be convincing enough to justify the policy change and investment (DesRoches et al., 2010). Therefore, the minimal clinically important difference (MCID) is imperative to consider in designing future studies.

Third, like other national sample surveys, MEPS experiences data missing owing to a series of logistic challenges, such as respondents' literacy limit, loss to follow-up, nonresponses and answers of "refused," "don't know," or other responses. Thus, we used substitution and complete case analyses to deal with these missings.

Fourth, although MEPS data is designed to be nationally representative, it does not include people who were institutionalized, in the military or homeless. Therefore, the populations being excluded may lead to underestimates and limit the generalizability of findings for those groups who have higher rates of chronic conditions.

Fifth, due to the limit of secondary data, the measure of PCC status in our study is operationalized form the existed variables regarding patient's perspective rather than researcher-initiated measures from primary data collection. So our study was limited by PCC measures available in the current collected dataset. Similarly, the limitations of outcome measures within MEPS preclude the examination of clinical or other more objective health outcomes. The MEPS data used in our study are mainly based on the patient' self-reported information, which would raise concerns of over-reporting or under-reporting the outcomes. Therefore, despite efforts to validate data, MEPS relies on a single household respondent's recall and is subject to recall bias, as they were asked to memorize their own and their family member's healthcare utilization.

Finally, although we have controlled for patient's predisposing, enabling, need factors and system covariates, our estimates may have been confounded by other unmeasured factors due to the limits of the nature of secondary data. One possible factor could be the severity of the disease, which was not be controlled due to no related variables available in MEPS. However, the severity or acuity of illness might explain why the PCC is not associated with the better outcome variable. The reason is that the patients with severe conditions would be more likely to receive PCC, and at the same time they would be more likely to experience hospitalization.

References

Ahmed, S., Berzon, R. A., Revicki, D. A., Lenderking, W. R., Moinpour, C. M., Basch, E., Reeve, B. B., Wu, A. W., & International Society for Quality of Life Research. (2012). The use of patient-reported outcomes (PRO) within comparative effectiveness research: Implications for clinical practice and health care policy. *Medical Care, 50*(12), 1060–1070.

Arend, J., Tsang-Quinn, J., Levine, C., & Thomas, D. (2012). The patient-centered medical home: History, components, and review of the evidence. *Mount Sinai Journal of Medicine, 79*(4), 433–450. https://doi.org/10.1002/msj.21326

Bakitas, M., Lyons, K. D., Hegel, M. T., Balan, S., Brokaw, F. C., Seville, J., Hull, J. G., Li, Z., Tosteson, T. D., Byock, I. R., & Ahles, T. A. (2009). Effects of a palliative care intervention on clinical outcomes in patients with advanced cancer: The project ENABLE II randomized controlled trial. *JAMA, 302*(7), 741–749.

Bechtel, C., & Ness, D. L. (2010). If you build it, will they come? Designing truly patient-centered health care. *Health Affairs (Millwood), 29*(5), 914–920.

Brownson, R. C., Gurney, J. G., & Land, G. H. (1999). Evidence-based decision making in public health. *Journal of Public Health Management and Practice, 5*(5), 86–97.

Calveley, J., Verhoeven, A., & Hopcroft, D. (2009). A patient-centred referral pathway for mild to moderate lifestyle and mental health problems: Does this model work in practice? *Journal of Primary Health Care, 1*(1), 50–56.

Carman, K. L., Dardess, P., Maurer, M., Sofaer, S., Adams, K., Bechtel, C., & Sweeney, J. (2013). Patient and family engagement: A framework for understanding the elements and developing interventions and policies. *Health Affairs (Millwood), 32*(2), 223–231.

Chung, A. E., & Basch, E. M. (2015). Incorporating the patient's voice into electronic health records through patient-reported outcomes as the "review of systems". *Journal of the American Medical Informatics Association, 22*(4), 914–916.

Coulter, A. (2012). Patient engagement—What works? *Journal of Ambulatory Care Management, 35*(2), 80–89.

Coulter, A., & Ellins, J. (2007). Effectiveness of strategies for informing, educating, and involving patients. *BMJ, 335*(7609), 24–27.

Crabtree, B. F., Nutting, P. A., Miller, W. L., Stange, K. C., Stewart, E. E., & Jaen, C. R. (2010). Summary of the national demonstration project and recommendations for the patient-centered medical home. *Annals of Family Medicine, 8*(Suppl 1), S80–S90, S92.

Cronholm, P. F., Shea, J. A., Werner, R. M., Miller-Day, M., Tufano, J., Crabtree, B. F., & Gabbay, R. (2013). The patient centered medical home: Mental models and practice culture driving the transformation process. *Journal of General Internal Medicine, 28*(9), 1195–1201.

DesRoches, C. M., Campbell, E. G., Vogeli, C., Zheng, J., Rao, S. R., Shields, A. E., Donelan, K., Rosenbaum, S., Bristol, S. J., & Jha, A. K. (2010). Electronic health records' limited successes suggest more targeted uses. *Health Affairs (Millwood), 29*(4), 639–646.

Ferrante, J. M., Balasubramanian, B. A., Hudson, S. V., & Crabtree, B. F. (2010). Principles of the patient-centered medical home and preventive services delivery. *Annals of Family Medicine, 8*(2), 108–116.

Flach, S. D., McCoy, K. D., Vaughn, T. E., Ward, M. M., Bootsmiller, B. J., & Doebbeling, B. N. (2004). Does patient-centered care improve provision of preventive services? *Journal of General Internal Medicine, 19*(10), 1019–1026.

Hibbard, J. H., & Greene, J. (2013). What the evidence shows about patient activation: Better health outcomes and care experiences; fewer data on costs. *Health Affairs (Millwood), 32*(2), 207–214.

Hillestad, R., Bigelow, J., Bower, A., Girosi, F., Meili, R., Scoville, R., & Taylor, R. (2005). Can electronic medical record systems transform health care? Potential health benefits, savings, and costs. *Health Affairs (Millwood), 24*(5), 1103–1117.

Jackson, G. L., Powers, B. J., Chatterjee, R., Bettger, J. P., Kemper, A. R., Hasselblad, V., Dolor, R. J., Irvine, R. J., Heidenfelder, B. L., Kendrick, A. S., Gray, R., & Williams, J. W. (2013). Improving patient care. The patient centered medical home. A systematic review. *Annals of Internal Medicine, 158*(3), 169–178.

Jencks, S. F., Williams, M. V., & Coleman, E. A. (2009). Rehospitalizations among patients in the Medicare fee-for-service program. *New England Journal of Medicine, 360*(14), 1418–1428.

Kahn, K. L., Schneider, E. C., Malin, J. L., Adams, J. L., & Epstein, A. M. (2007). Patient centered experiences in breast cancer: Predicting long-term adherence to tamoxifen use. *Medical Care, 45*(5), 431–439.

Kilo, C. M., & Wasson, J. H. (2010). Practice redesign and the patient-centered medical home: History, promises, and challenges. *Health Affairs (Millwood), 29*(5), 773–778.

Leibowitz, R., Day, S., & Dunt, D. (2003). A systematic review of the effect of different models of after-hours primary medical care services on clinical outcome, medical workload, and patient and GP satisfaction. *Family Practice, 20*(3), 311–317.

Link, B. G., Northridge, M. E., Phelan, J. C., & Ganz, M. L. (1998). Social epidemiology and the fundamental cause concept: On the structuring of effective cancer screens by socioeconomic status. *Milbank Quarterly, 76*(3), 375–402, 304–305.

Lohr, K. N., & Zebrack, B. J. (2009). Using patient-reported outcomes in clinical practice: Challenges and opportunities. *Quality of Life Research, 18*(1), 99–107.

Markovitz, A. R., Alexander, J. A., Lantz, P. M., & Paustian, M. L. (2015). Patient-centered medical home implementation and use of preventive services: The role of practice socioeconomic context. *JAMA Internal Medicine, 175*(4), 598–606.

Michie, S., Abraham, C., Whittington, C., McAteer, J., & Gupta, S. (2009). Effective techniques in healthy eating and physical activity interventions: A meta-regression. *Health Psychology, 28*(6), 690–701.

Moore, A. D., Hamilton, J. B., Pierre-Louis, B. J., & Jennings, B. M. (2013). Increasing access to care and reducing mistrust: Important considerations when implementing the patient-centered medical home in army health clinics. *Military Medicine, 178*(3), 291–298.

Morey, J. C., Simon, R., Jay, G. D., Wears, R. L., Salisbury, M., Dukes, K. A., & Berns, S. D. (2002). Error reduction and performance improvement in the emergency department through

formal teamwork training: Evaluation results of the MedTeams project. *Health Services Research, 37*(6), 1553–1581.
Murray, M., & Berwick, D. M. (2003). Advanced access: Reducing waiting and delays in primary care. *JAMA, 289*(8), 1035–1040.
Nelson, K. M., Helfrich, C., Sun, H., Hebert, P. L., Liu, C. F., Dolan, E., Taylor, L., Wong, E., Maynard, C., Hernandez, S. E., Sanders, W., Randall, I., Curtis, I., Schectman, G., Stark, R., & Fihn, S. D. (2014). Implementation of the patient-centered medical home in the veterans health administration: Associations with patient satisfaction, quality of care, staff burnout, and hospital and emergency department use. *JAMA Internal Medicine, 174*(8), 1350–1358.
Nutting, P. A., Miller, W. L., Crabtree, B. F., Jaen, C. R., Stewart, E. E., & Stange, K. C. (2009). Initial lessons from the first national demonstration project on practice transformation to a patient-centered medical home. *Annals of Family Medicine, 7*(3), 254–260.
O'Connell, J. M., Stanley, J. L., & Malakar, C. L. (2001). Satisfaction and patient outcomes of a telephone-based nurse triage service. *Managed Care, 10*(7), 55–56, 59–60, 65.
O'Malley, A. S., Beaton, E., Yabroff, K. R., Abramson, R., & Mandelblatt, J. (2004). Patient and provider barriers to colorectal cancer screening in the primary care safety-net. *Preventive Medicine, 39*(1), 56–63.
Ortman, J. M., Velkoff, V. A., & Hogan, H. (2014). An aging nation: The older population in the United States, current population reports. Accessed January 8, 2016. Available at: https://www.census.gov/prod/2014pubs/p25-1140.pdf
Radwin, L. E., Cabral, H. J., & Woodworth, T. S. (2013). Effects of race and language on patient-centered cancer nursing care and patient outcomes. *Journal of Health Care for the Poor and Underserved, 24*(2), 619–632.
Reid, R. J., Fishman, P. A., Yu, O., Ross, T. R., Tufano, J. T., Soman, M. P., & Larson, E. B. (2009). Patient-centered medical home demonstration: A prospective, quasi-experimental, before and after evaluation. *The American Journal of Managed Care, 15*(9), e71–e87.
Reid, R. J., Coleman, K., Johnson, E. A., Fishman, P. A., Hsu, C., Soman, M. P., Trescott, C. E., Erikson, M., & Larson, E. B. (2010). The group health medical home at year two: Cost savings, higher patient satisfaction, and less burnout for providers. *Health Affairs (Millwood), 29*(5), 835–843.
Roberts, K. J. (2002). Physician-patient relationships, patient satisfaction, and antiretroviral medication Adherence among HIV-infected adults attending a public health clinic. *AIDS Patient Care and STDs, 16*(1), 43–50.
Roter, D. L., Stashefsky-Margalit, R., & Rudd, R. (2001). Current perspectives on patient education in the US. *Patient Education and Counseling, 44*(1), 79–86.
Salyers, M. P., Matthias, M. S., Spann, C. L., Lydick, J. M., Rollins, A. L., & Frankel, R. M. (2009). The role of patient activation in psychiatric visits. *Psychiatric Services (Washington, D. C.), 60*(11), 1535–1539.
Sarfaty, M., Wender, R., & Smith, R. (2011). Promoting cancer screening within the patient centered medical home. *CA: A Cancer Journal for Clinicians, 61*(6), 397–408.
Stange, K. C. (2009). The problem of fragmentation and the need for integrative solutions. *Annals of Family Medicine, 7*(2), 100–103.
Stewart, M., Brown, J. B., Donner, A., McWhinney, I. R., Oates, J., Weston, W. W., & Jordan, J. (2000). The impact of patient-centered care on outcomes. *Journal of Family Practice, 49*(9), 796–804.
Tinetti, M. E., & Fried, T. (2004). The end of the disease era. *American Journal of Medicine, 116*(3), 179–185.
Valderas, J. M., Kotzeva, A., Espallargues, M., Guyatt, G., Ferrans, C. E., Halyard, M. Y., Revicki, D. A., Symonds, T., Parada, A., & Alonso, J. (2008). The impact of measuring patient-reported outcomes in clinical practice: A systematic review of the literature. *Quality of Life Research, 17*(2), 179–193.

Wagner, P. J., Dias, J., Howard, S., Kintziger, K. W., Hudson, M. F., Seol, Y. H., & Sodomka, P. (2012). Personal health records and hypertension control: A randomized trial. *Journal of the American Medical Informatics Association, 19*(4), 626–634.

Waxmonsky, J. A., Giese, A. A., McGinnis, G. F., Reynolds, R. T., Abrahamson, A., McKitterick, M. L., Coleman, L., & Thomas, M. R. (2011). Colorado access' enhanced care management for high-cost, high-need Medicaid members: Preliminary outcomes and lessons learned. *Journal of Ambulatory Care Management, 34*(2), 183–191.

Williams, G. C., Lynch, M., & Glasgow, R. E. (2007). Computer-assisted intervention improves patient-centered diabetes care by increasing autonomy support. *Health Psychology, 26*(6), 728–734.

Wu, A. W., Kharrazi, H., Boulware, L. E., & Snyder, C. F. (2013). Measure once, cut twice—Adding patient-reported outcome measures to the electronic health record for comparative effectiveness research. *Journal of Clinical Epidemiology, 66*(8 Suppl), S12–S20.

Yedidia, M. J. (2007). Transforming doctor-patient relationships to promote patient-centered care: Lessons from palliative care. *Journal of Pain and Symptom Management, 33*(1), 40–57.

Zolnierek, K. B., & Dimatteo, M. R. (2009). Physician communication and patient adherence to treatment: A meta-analysis. *Medical Care, 47*(8), 826–834.

Chapter 9
Conclusion

The findings that demonstrate the associations between PCC status and health process as well as outcome measures argues for added efforts to examine the order of the events and to establish the causality by using quasi-experiment and even experiment study designs. Given the feasible, ethical and affordable considerations of study design, rigorous quasi-experiments are specifically poised to generate estimates that can be brought to bear in clinical decision making and government policy making (Greenfield & Platt, 2012). Future studies may also consider measuring both gain in health from a PCC intervention and the cost associated with the health gain to estimate the potential cost-effectiveness of PCC program aimed at chronic condition management among older adults. Emphasis on such rigorous research designs would be helpful in reporting results in terms of statistical significance as well as clinical significance, and therefore efficiently convincing policy makers to investment more efforts and resources on scaling-up PCC strategies. At the same time, ethical considerations are as important as the economic and effective judgements in advocate of the PCC. Future studies should also be explore the promise of and concerns about the PCC through the lens of ethics.

Additional studies could also include practice and provider level data for investigating the relationship between PCC characteristics and the health process as well as outcome measures. For example, we could compare the acute inpatient admission rates between PCC and non-PCC patient groups by using practice-level longitudinal claims data from elderly Medicare patients who attend the primary care facilities over a period of time. The findings from such study could demonstrate the long-term and sustainable impact of PCC on the improvements in patient health outcomes and the quality of care.

Moreover, further consensus, development, validation and refinement of PCC measures for elderly chronic patients are imperative and should become a future research priority. The reason is because the most existing evaluation measures and tools are mainly designed for all the patient population. However, not only patients but also providers and governors need valid and meaningful information to accurately evaluate PCC for the elderly chronic patients and allocate relevant resources for them.

H. Liang, *The Impact of Patient-Centered Care*,
https://doi.org/10.1007/978-981-16-3968-5_9

Future researches are needed to development new evaluation tools or to adapt existing tools to make the evaluation more suitable and valid for the specific group of users.

Although our study have linked PCC status and its individual attributes to health process and outcome variables, further research is needed to investigate how process variables are related to outcomes within each PCC subgroup, and examine what organizational arrangements are optimal in providing these PCC components. Such researches can help explain the nature of PCC, so that the limited resources can be allocated effectively. Future analyses could also include more objective and salient outcome variables, such as the patient's physical and clinical data to examine the health outcomes among older adults with specific chronic conditions (Rittenhouse et al., 2010).

Furthermore, additional studies that focus on how PCC could improve care for patients with complex needs are needed. Not only chronic care, future research could also focus on PCC that could be extended beyond just chronic illness but conditions that require long-term care. With the population aging and more people living longer with chronic conditions, the demand for long-term care services will explode in present-day and near-future. Our study shows promise of PCC for older adults with chronic conditions, additional studies can be conducted to investigate if PCC is applicable to any patient population with long-term care needs.

The overall goal of this book was to improve understandings of the relationship between the PCC and the receipt of selected preventive services as well as the patient's health outcomes in the United States. The study highlights the impact of PCC on the elderly chronic disease patients' health experiences, process of care, and health outcomes. The study adds to the evidence that PCC is associated with better performance in delivering care to the elderly with significant burden of chronic conditions in the United States. Our study is unique in the measures' comprehensiveness, and therefore adding solid support that the implementation of PCC model is associated with better health care performance.

Seeking to improve the chronic care for all patients, ethics of care and current care imperatives are leading us in the direction of advocating for policies that supports the improvement efforts of PCC. The findings of our study also show the impact of each of the three attributes of PCC on the health process and outcome measures, and the results furtherly inform the three components of PCC—the whole person care, the patient engagement and the enhanced access—are highly interdependent. Along with the evidence from in-depth research on the impact of essential components as well as the whole model of PCC, policy makers should adopt appropriate models/components of PCC to achieve more remarkable performance in older patients' chronic care (Nutting et al., 2009). A better understanding of the fundamental determinants of chronic care quality may help point to effective policies and strategies to improve care, and health outcomes among our targeted elderly population with chronic conditions. Researchers need continue to investigate the optimal care model to cope with the current demographic transition and the shifting burden of disease, which furtherly will inform policy makers to strengthen healthcare systems, improve population well-being and address health disparities in the United States.

References

Greenfield, S., & Platt, R. (2012). Can observational studies approximate RCTs? *Value Health, 15*(2), 215–216.

Nutting, P. A., Miller, W. L., Crabtree, B. F., Jaen, C. R., Stewart, E. E., & Stange, K. C. (2009). Initial lessons from the first national demonstration project on practice transformation to a patient-centered medical home. *Annals of Family Medicine, 7*(3), 254–260.

Rittenhouse, D. R., Thom, D. H., & Schmittdiel, J. A. (2010). Developing a policy-relevant research agenda for the patient-centered medical home: A focus on outcomes. *Journal of General Internal Medicine, 25*(6), 593–600.

The manufacturer's authorised representative in the EU is Springer Nature Customer Service Centre GmbH, Europaplatz 3, 69115 Heidelberg, Germany. If you have any concerns regarding our products, please contact ProductSafety@springernature.com

Printed and bound by CPI Group (UK) Ltd, Croydon, CR0 4YY
30/09/2026
02225264-0008